Conversations
with
Breast Cancer Patients

Conversations
with
Breast Cancer Patients

~ ~ ~ ~ ~ ~ ~ ~ ~ ~ ~ ~ ~ ~ ~ ~ ~ ~

Revised Edition 2015

Ernest Greenberg, MD

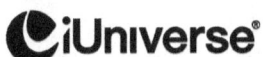

Conversations with Breast Cancer Patients

Writers Advantage
an imprint of iUniverse, Inc.

iUniverse books may be ordered through booksellers or by contacting:

iUniverse
1663 Liberty Drive
Bloomington, IN 47403
www.iuniverse.com
1-800-Authors (1-800-288-4677)

ISBN: 978-0-5952-5943-4 (sc)
ISBN: 978-0-5956-5452-9 (hc)

Print information available on the last page.

iUniverse rev. date: 07/22/2015

QUOTATIONS

Some patients clearly are alive and disease-free a decade or more after initial relapse. The fraction may be small, but the accomplishment is not. The patient with metastatic breast cancer is in a desperate but not uniformly hopeless situation. Perhaps we might, in the not too distant future, expand this message of hope to the majority of patients with metastatic breast cancer. To do so will probably require something quite different from today's combination chemotherapy. But the dream is not an impossible one.

George W. Sledge
Editorial. Cancer 14:2191, August 1996

En médecine comme en amour ni jamais ni toujours.
(In medicine as in love neither say "never" nor "always".)

French saying, anonymous.

You gotta a-ccen-tuate the positive
E-li-minate the negative.

Johnny Mercer (lyrics)

ACKNOWLEDGEMENT

Two physicians have been greatly instrumental in guiding my professional life in the field of investigation and treatment of breast cancer. One of them was Dr. Olof Pearson who offered me a fellowship in his research section at the Sloan-Kettering Cancer Institute. The other was Dr. Paul Juret of the Institut Gustave-Roussy in Paris who, at that time, visited the Center periodically and became a close friend. Over the years and during our many visits across the ocean we shared our experiences in treating *the patients* harboring this disease. This book is dedicated to their memory.

This work, relating some of my experiences in my life as an oncologist was made possible thanks to my wife Anna who stood by while I cared for others, who waited long hours in our car while I stopped at the hospital, at the office, or at a patient's home while we missed the openings of operas, concerts or plays, were late for dinner appointments, and put large segments of our life on hold. She supported and encouraged me in my endeavor to write this book, brought back events to my memory, read and re-read my manuscript and reassured me when I felt it did not meet the standard or the purpose I had assigned to it. When she herself was struck with breast cancer she opened for me a personal window of understanding of the physical and the emotional consequences of that diagnosis and of its treatment.

I also wish to recall the joy afforded by my sons Marc and Paul who, as children, got out of bed when I came home at eleven every night, in order to keep me company as I sat for very late dinners. They sensed, in spite of the personal strain, the satisfaction and excitement of practicing medicine and have both become skilled and compassionate physicians.

I wish to thank my friend Edith Ratshin for her patience in reading and help in correcting and editing the first edition of Conversations with Breast Cancer Patients.

This work is also dedicated to all those courageous women and men who, facing the burden of their cancer, came to me for advice and care, and in the process, taught me about their lives and their struggles. In the course of this they contributed immensely to the maturation of the way I thought about and adjusted to having to face those persons whose lives were often threatened by fatal illness.

CONTENTS

PREFACE TO THE SECOND EDITION

The reader of this book has to be mindful of the fact that the conversations that are related in it have taken place in most part at a time before the advent of genetic testing and identification of markers of risk such as BRCA-1, BRCA-2, HER2 and others presently still being evaluated. Since that time the observations of different combinations of hormone receptors and genetic markers in tumor tissues have found their place as risk and prognostic determinants of the course of breast cancers. These observations have led to the design of a new classification system for this malignancy. The identification of these risk-connected gene abnormalities has been a landmark development. Genetic testing for such factors has become one of the most promising fields in identifying risk factors yet unknown as well as vulnerability to specific treatments.

Since the first edition of Conversations with Breast Cancer patients many changes have taken place in the spectrum of breast cancer and in its management. It has become increasingly evident that breast cancer represents a group of malignancies of that organ with different susceptibilities to treatment modalities and different clinical courses. The spectrum of the disease has changed as a result of improvements in diagnosis, in the development of newer treatment programs and of better strategies targeting the cancerous tissue. Along with these, and with the identification of specific risk factors, prevention has been making inroads. Immunotherapy, a field that is still undergoing active investigation, will open the way to a totally different form of treatment and possibly prevention.

Both earlier diagnosis and, as a result, patients presenting with much smaller cancers than in the past have led to a marked decrease in the need for mastectomy. This as well as the improvement in the methods of breast reconstruction, has decreased the fear of the disfigurement associated with this procedure and women are seeking prompt medical advice for breast problems. In addition, the fact that it is increasingly common to start or to prepare for the process of reconstruction at the time of the mastectomy has diminished the concerns of patients about the post-surgical deformity of the chest.

That is not to say that the fear of cancer is no longer strong in the mind of those diagnosed with this disease. The questions of why it happened, whether to treat, when to treat, how to treat and what happens without treatment, are still asked. The questions of how to live with the disease and its treatment and of how long one is expected to survive are ever present and must be addressed by the treating physician when they are raised. Palliative care all along and terminal care are issues that are increasingly recognized as part of the ongoing care of the patient.

The "C" word is out of the closet and physicians have, for the most part, become more comfortable in discussing it with their patients, acknowledging its seriousness while emphasizing hope. Hope in its various forms, a most important topic, is addressed very specifically, in one of the related conversations. In this revision referrals to specific chemotherapeutic agents by name have been deliberately avoided because the purpose of this book is not to provide information about the constantly and rapidly changing medications in use or how and when to use them. Its purpose is to present the reader with an understanding of the feelings of the person facing the challenge and the threat of a potentially fatal illness, its treatment and about how that person's interaction with his or her physician may help navigated the stormy waters ahead. Likewise hormonal therapy, an important part of the armamentarium used against breast cancer, is mentioned repeatedly in the text without identifying its particular form by name. Yet it is explained that some forms of hormonal interventions are very effective in the treatment of breast cancer while others, different ones, may stimulate its growth. The conversations remain unchanged in this edition although the analysis of their contents has sometimes been expanded in keeping with the growing understanding of the disease.

It is my hope that this revised edition will continue to help improve communication between physicians and their patients by concentrating on the needs of the person as well as on the treatment of the illness she or he is harboring. While it has focused mainly on actual conversations with breast cancer patients it relates as well to many of the problems of those afflicted with other cancers. In many of the sections of this book I dwell on the role of the patient in the decision making regarding the treatment plan. I believe that a well-informed patient is a partner in this process. Treatment is offered not imposed. It is also my view that the physician who has periodically given thought about personally confronting the many issues facing the patients seeking answers, including contemplating the time nearing death, would be better prepared to answer these questions.

Ernest Greenberg, MD
June 22, 2015

PREFACE TO THE FIRST EDITION

During more than forty years devoted for the most part to the treatment of women as well as of some men afflicted with breast cancer, and to the study of this condition, I have seen most if not all the variations in the course of this malignancy, witnessed the reactions of these people to their illness and to its treatment, and observed the many ways in which it influenced and modified their lives and their relationships. Most of all, I have been overwhelmed by the courage with which the women faced their bodily changes, the discomfort of their treatment and, for so many of them, the ravages caused by this cancer.

More importantly, I have witnessed over these years the progress that has taken place in the methods of early diagnosis and early treatment of breast cancer for the purpose of increasing the rate of cure. I have also witnessed the progress in the methods of treatment of the advanced stages of this disease, and in the management of the uncomfortable symptoms associated with it and with its treatment. At the same time, preventive methods against it are emerging as a result of a growing understanding of risk factors as well as of the genetic and environmental antecedents that determine them.

I started practicing this field of medicine at a time when the word cancer was uttered in whispers and almost exclusively among physicians. It was hardly ever given as a diagnosis to a patient, neither was there any meaningful discussion of its impact on any aspect of that person's life.

Being slow by nature and consequently very patient I took the time to listen as people spoke when they came for their consultations, their treatments and their periodic follow up examinations. In the course of this process I also participated in the first program of open discussion about end of life attitudes for our hospital staff. I also started the first patients' group discussion about how to live with the problems of this cancer and its treatment. Through this process I learned a great deal from them. I learned what and how I could talk to them about their illness and its treatment. I learned how to listen to the cues they gave me, cues that helped me to inform and advise them in an acceptable, frank and yet non-threatening way. They taught me how people think when their health and their life are in serious jeopardy and how this in turn affects their personal relationships and attitudes, at times for the better and sometimes for the worst. I have witnessed the effects of that illness on their everyday lives, the reactions of their families, of their close friends, of their business associates as well as of some of their physicians.

This education on the job has enabled me to apply the knowledge I acquired, along with the constantly updated medical information, not only to treat them but just as importantly, to communicate with them. These conversations starting with their medical problems provided a means to hear about and to relieve their fears, to listen to their personal problems and dilemmas and to help them resolve them or live with them, to hear their wishes, their dreams, their plans, their fear of planning, their regrets, their hopes, their hopelessness, their fights, guide them to their victories and also sustain them through their surrenders. I think and hope that as a result of the medical care I provided and through these conversations I have been able to relieve their physical as well as their frequently overlooked emotional burdens. It has been a long voyage we took together each time, whether through calm or stormy weather.

The verbal interchange between patient and physician is the most important tool in the diagnosis of any illness and its complications. It is the most valuable one in evaluation the state of health of a person. It is the first line of investigation of the condition of the patient and it frequently determines the direction to follow in order to arrive at the definitive diagnosis. It is the major way by which the person who is ill conveys to the physician the extent to which the illness has affected his or her life. It is also the major avenue for the physician to explain the mechanism of the illness, to describe the treatment, to communicate to that person the reassurance that a treatment is undertaken that, hopefully, will relieve suffering and improve health.

It is for this reason that, for this book, I chose the format of a series of conversations, all of which having actually taken place, most of them many times with different persons facing the same problems. While the names are entirely fictitious and the circumstances in the text have been altered they are truly representative of the subjects discussed and the content of these exchanges is real. Many of these conversations also provided easily understandable explanations of the disease process in response to questions raised at the time as well as of the thought process leading to the recommendations about its treatments. It also is my hope that the reader, be he or she a physician or not, a healthy person or one having been marked by breast cancer, will find constructive, positive and helpful thoughts in them.

Since our understanding of the genesis, the evolution and the treatment of breast cancer are constantly expanding this book was not written as another primer on how to treat it because *treatment methods are constantly changing, frequently at only few months' intervals.* It was conceived mostly as a framework about how one can *live* with this illness and its treatment. It is based upon the personal experiences of many of those who have gone through that process, over a period of forty years. Its format is such that it has no formal continuity. While they may be grouped under a set of general headings each of these conversations covers a single question or a topic. Each one may be read out of the context of the entire book and therefore the reader may open it and read any part of it without necessarily having to follow a sequence of chapters.

This work also represents my own journey through the multiple phases of breast cancer in the company of the many patients I have treated over a period of more than forty years. At one end of that journey some have quickly reached a safe harbor and were able to settle down and shed their worry about the cancer at that time. Others have traveled with me without ever reaching the final destination of the cure and were lost sooner or later in the storm. Some remain aboard and are still going forth years later. I hope that this work will bring not only an understanding of how breast cancer behaves clinically but, as importantly, an understanding of the person who harbors that cancer and the awareness that relationships exist between the disease, its host and that host's other relationships in life. Above all, it is meant to emphasize the fact that life can and does go on for those who have been affected by this illness that the probability of cure is a reality and the possibility of eventual prevention is no longer in the realm of fantasy.

E.G.

SECTION I
AT FIRST

****

In this day and age, with the high degree of emphasis placed on physical beauty, health, and sexuality, particularly in the Western world, the finding of a breast lump is one of the most dreaded events a woman can experience at any age but particularly in the prime of her life, and worse even at a young age.

The thoughts first engendered by this finding are reflections of the traditional fear of cancer compounded by the stories heard, the news and books read, the movies or video programs seen, frequently depicting the worst possible scenarios associated with the diagnosis of breast cancer. These media never dwell upon the many who, having been diagnosed and treated for breast cancer, are cured and go on with the rest of their life. We are given scenarios of the fear and suffering, not the successes.

While not minimizing the potential seriousness, with emphasis on "potential," of the finding of a breast lump, I must immediately qualify such a finding by reminding the reader of the fact that the breast is frequently, to a greater or lesser extent, a "lumpy" organ and that fortunately many of its lumps are benign and physiological. That does not mean that such a lump may be safely overlooked but that immediate panic is not necessarily justified. It is also a fact that with the present and constantly improving diagnostic technology it has become possible to detect breast cancers of minuscule size and at a stage of development at which immediate and appropriate treatment is associated with a very high rate of permanent *CURE*. Indeed, over the past several years the mortality from breast cancer finally stabilized and then declined while it had been rising for a long time in the past. At present questions are even raised about the true significance of the very tiny cancerous or pre-cancerous lesions detected by the ever increasing improvement of the mammographic images obtained by the ever increasing technological precision of the diagnostic equipment: should every single one of these increasingly smaller lesions be followed by biopsy and / or excision?

Surgery for breast cancer has become progressively less extensive and even in circumstances under which the breast has to be removed by mastectomy, the surgical technique of breast reconstruction has evolved to the point where physical appearance can be restored to a degree that also restores the self-image of the woman who has had to undergo that type of cancer surgery. On the other hand, a growing proportion of the women with breast cancer do not have to lose the affected breast because the increasingly early detection of cancers generally smaller than in the past, makes it possible to preserve it, thus avoiding the disfigurement of mastectomy. Furthermore, while the addition of radiation therapy to breast-conserving surgery, as an integral part of the initial treatment, has resulted in long-term outcomes identical to those of the previous standard mastectomy, it is not without certain long delayed after-effects including the rare development of other malignancies related to the radiation.

Finally, chemotherapy and/or hormonal therapy administered as part of the initial management (adjuvant systemic therapy) of breast cancer, when indicated, have improved both the survival and the cure rate for this malignancy. For the women for whom it is indicated the contemplation of having to undergo months of administration of these medications after the initial more or less extensive surgery and radiation therapy for some, is certainly disruptive and many of the media depictions and publicized personal stories have emphasized the frightening and uncomfortable aspects of this category of treatments. It is therefore not unexpected that its application is contemplated with dread. Yet, just as progress in the techniques of surgery, radiation, plastic reconstruction and chemotherapy has improved the quality of their results, new developments have improved the supportive measures designed not only to relieve but also to prevent the uncomfortable side effects of this chemotherapy, to the point that they seldom cause any serious disruption of the life and wellbeing of its recipients. Again, as with radiation therapy, certain long delayed complications are increasingly being recognized.

I have also found that the most devastating side effect of chemotherapy is not the nausea, the fatigue, the metabolic or hormonal changes, but it is the difficult-to-hide loss of hair. While that is the least medically important one and while it is temporary, it is, for a woman, other than the loss of a breast, the side effect that is associated with the greatest emotional impact, one that cannot be minimized and that has to be acknowledged and dealt with: the further disruption of the self-image.

In this section the story titled "This is New York" depicts one person's way of dealing with that feature of her disrupted physical appearance. Her story is unique and personal and only serves to illustrate the fact that each individual finds his or her way of dealing with that problem. It is frequently the attitude of those surrounding and interacting with the main character of this personal drama, that requires correction, guidance, and help, help that often comes from the patient herself.

The effects of the entire complex system including the diagnosis, the treatment, the profound and invisible physiological changes it produces as well as the emotional impact of it all on the woman herself, on those closest to her and on her sexuality, are frequently unmentioned and overlooked in her day-to-day care because they either are not physically obvious to the observing physician, because the patient feels uncomfortable complaining about these problems or because the physician is not prepared to deal with them. This complex after-shock associated with the treatment and course of this illness impacts on the lives on many of the involved couples because it has to do in good part with sexuality and because the problems of one member of these couples also impact the other. They should be addressed as an integral part of the patient's medical management. The recipient of the treatment should be made to feel that these problems can be addressed comfortably and candidly in the physician's office. While some may have to be referred for care by another specialist the existence of this profound impact on their life should at least be recognized and must be addressed.

Guilt, unexplained, undeserved and frequently self-imposed, is a burden many women carry once diagnosed. Such guilt can be relieved by reassurance and explanations lest it becomes an additional source of unnecessary emotional anguish.

Some of these feelings and questions brought up by women recently diagnosed with breast cancer are illustrated in the conversations related in this section. No one can convey them better than those immediately involved, the woman herself, her closest ones, spouse, family, friend or lover, and her physician.

THE LUMP

The journey through breast cancer often starts with the "lump."

Alice was forty-eight and, because of her family history of breast cancer, she had come for her yearly breast examination and mammograms since the age of forty. She had called for an appointment one month ahead of her scheduled yearly visit because she had found a lump in her left breast that morning.

Now she sat in my small consultation room in the only available armchair not yet overtaken by the mounting stacks of mail and medical journals. The two glass cabinets hanging on the wall behind her were the only truly neat havens in that space. They contain various small gifts presented to me over the years by people I have cared for. My favorite is the ivory Chinese "medicine doll" in the cabinet on my left as I look at that wall. The story I was told is that in the high social circles of ancient China women did not leave their homes, not even to visit their physician. They would send instead one of their ladies-in-waiting carrying a carved ivory representation of a reclining woman. The messenger would indicate to the physician the part of the body that was the source of her mistress' distress. Based on that information, the physician would then prescribe the remedy, potion or poultice he deemed appropriate to treat the illness. I frequently wondered as I would sometimes stop in the course of the day and gaze at that elegant reclining white shape of a woman with her eternal and mysterious smile, how the female patients with breast lumps fared under that system of health care delivery. The practice of medicine has certainly become more complex since then.

"So, Doctor... what do you think of this lump?" asked Alice.

Her tone was both casual and concerned. It was the tone of someone truly worried but not wanting to make much of something that, while it might not deserve that much concern in the long run, was nevertheless a source of considerable anxiety reflected in her eyes and her entire body attitude at that particular time.

I had tried to be reassuring without being casual although a woman who comes to consult me about a lump in her breast is always a cause for concern. I tried to keep my face from showing any worry but this is a difficult task. A blank face is not a reassuring one because I do not ordinarily keep a blank face. A smile was not appropriate. I decided simply to express what I felt.

"It is there all right," I told her. "I can feel it easily but I cannot tell for sure whether it is truly a tumor or a bunch of cysts since your breast contains many smaller lumps that feel almost the same as this one and have always been there. I did not make any mention of this one in the notes of your last examination and therefore I think it is new although not necessarily serious. By the way, when do you expect to have your next period?"

She relaxed a little.

"In about two weeks. My breasts are starting to feel a little swollen but this...thing feels different to me."

I knew what she meant. It felt different to me too, not out-and-out sinister, as I put it sometimes, but prominent enough to be worrisome and reason enough to be sure to check further into its nature.

I told her that he best would be for her to have a set of mammograms and then decide what else to do. "You would be due for it next month anyway," I added.

"So you think it is cancerous," she persisted.

"That is not what I said. Cancer is of course the thing I have to think of first but the diagnosis has to be obtained in the appropriate way. Sometimes it is immediately obvious. In your case it is not. Let me take the time to check it fully as soon as possible before jumping to a conclusion."

"When should I have the mammogram done?" she asked.

Her heart rate during the examination had told me how scared she had truly been. I picked up the telephone.

"I already called to find out if they will take you now or later today. This way I will be able to tell you more without having you sitting on hot coals over the weekend."

Now while she was worried she had at least the feeling that no time was being lost. She knew that although I had tried to reassure her I was concerned enough myself to try to speed up the process of determining the nature of that lump.

"Tell me... should I worry?"

"Can I tell you not to?" I replied. "That is why I am trying to resolve this today. What can I say? Don't worry too much now. Let us deal with facts and not build sinister fancies until these facts are available. Go to Dr. Gordon now, you know his office. They are expecting you."

"Yes, but I must call my husband to have him meet me there when I have the mammogram. I don't feel I can face this alone. Oh my God! I am so scared doctor!"

"I know and I think it is a good idea to call your husband. You may then both come back here with your mammograms after Dr. Gordon has seen them and talked to me. We will then discuss the findings and what to do about them if anything."

"I am terribly scared."

Her older sister and one of her maternal aunts had died of breast cancer and that is how she had come to my office several years earlier when she would accompany them for their treatment and follow up. That is also why she eventually decided to come at regular intervals for breast examinations in addition to her yearly mammograms and breast self-examination which she had been instructed to perform monthly. It was already known that breast cancer could be frequent in certain families but the genetic* abnormalities associated with such "familial" breast cancer had not yet been discovered at that time.

"I know. Go and come back."

I could not help being anxious myself about this. Over the years, a various times, I have taken care of several members of a family for treatment breast cancer. It was either a sister or a daughter or a mother of the one who had originally come to me. Each time this happens my inner reaction is the feeling that I am experiencing the relapse of a serious illness that I am unable to shake completely. It is as if I have to undergo treatment all over again. On one occasion several years ago, seeing my reaction to the call of another member of such a family my wife tried to dissuade me from taking on her case.

Two hours later Alice returned with her husband.

"Hello Mr. Filipides, Mrs. Filipides. Please sit down." I had cleared the other chair of all the paper stuff, which had covered it, letters, publications, notices of new regulations, advertisements, and professional journals... "Show me the films. I spoke with Dr. Gordon already."

I placed the films on the X-ray viewing box and examined them.

"As you already know he not only did the regular mammograms but he also took magnified views of the spot we are all concerned about as well as an ultrasound examination. He finds nothing suspicious on these studies. Yet you do have this somewhat thickened area in the breast on examination. Having looked at all the films myself I am satisfied of the fact that I also find nothing corresponding to the area of thickening that is causing all of us to worry."

"So, where do we go from here?"

"Some cancers, fortunately few, do not show up on the mammogram and more so in younger women because the breast tissue is dense and relatively opaque to x-ray. Since you have a family history of breast cancer, I feel that I should be particularly careful in your situation. I think it is a good idea for you to return here for a recheck of the breast shortly after your next period. If I can still feel the same thickened area at that time, I think a biopsy will be indicated to start with. What follows will depend upon the findings. If the biopsy is negative, I would still repeat the mammogram in four to five months just to make sure everything is OK."

"What if the biopsy shows it is cancer Doctor?"

I have had to deal with "what if" all my professional life. "What if(s)" cannot be brushed off.

"We shall cross this bridge if or when we meet it and hope we don't. Since we have not met it yet there is no point in creating an entire scenario about something that does not exists and live in fear prematurely and unnecessarily. I know this is not easy and I wish there were a better way to handle it but there is not."

As it turned out the questionable breast lump had disappeared by the time she returned for the follow up examination two weeks later, after her period was over. She was so relieved she cried. I was relieved too. There is the cliché that people tell their physician: "Oh! You must be immune to all these problems that you see." No, I am not immune to the anxiety and the suffering of the patient. I may not show it but I feel it day after day and I have known some colleagues who changed their specialty from their oncology practice because unable to sustain the constant stress and anxiety associated with it. My answer to this comment is that the victories won in the course of treating people suffering from cancer amply make up for the heartache of the defeats. The fact is that cancer treatment is a field of medicine in which changes and progress occur at such a rapid rate that hopes for greater victories sustain physicians and patients alike.

Several years ago, one of my typists resigned her position in my office because she could no longer emotionally bear transcribing the histories and clinical follow up notes of women she did not even know and never saw. Hospital nurses have many times sought relief of the emotional stress associated with the care of cancer patients through psychological counseling provided at their institution.

As for Alice, this had been an unavoidable fright and fortunately only a fright! She never embarked on the journey and remains well to this day.

I DID NOT KNOW THAT MEN...

"I did not know that men could also have breast cancer."

Fred had been referred to me for chemotherapy after having undergone a right mastectomy for breast cancer. The cancer had been found to be locally extensive with most of the lymph nodes removed at surgery already invaded by the cancer.

"Yes it does happen." I explained that since men have breasts, as under-developed as they may be, they can get breast cancer. Its frequency is much smaller than for women there being one male breast cancer for every hundred breast cancers in women and they behave generally the same way in both.

"When I found out I could not believe it," he said. "How could this happen to me? Then I did a computer search. I looked it up and I found out that its course is usually worse in men than in women. How can it happen? Why?"

Fred was really upset. Not only he had a cancer but he had a woman's cancer. In our still male dominated society this was what is known as a "double whammy."

"Men can get breast cancer in the tiny amount of breast tissue they normally have. But it is not worse in men. The reason why breast cancer *seems* to have a more serious course in males is that it is frequently diagnosed at a more advanced stage. Unfortunately, many physicians do not routinely examine men's breasts for lumps and when a lump is found it is frequently overlooked for a long time both by the physician and by the man himself. The result is that often by the time such a lump is finally biopsied, diagnosed, and definitive surgery is performed the disease is often already advanced and its prognosis from then on is more serious."

"This is exactly what happened to me. I noted the tiny lump in my left breast more than a year ago. It was very small, did not bother me and I did not do anything about it. When I showed it to my family physician a few months ago he felt it but thought nothing of it. It is only when I mentioned it to my tennis partner and to his son who is a radiologist, while we were in the locker room of our club, that he told me to come for a mammogram. I had it done the following day and he promptly referred me to a breast surgeon. That is truly how the cancer was found. If we had not all three been in the club's locker room at the same time I would still be going around with my cancer. Fortunately it has been found and has been removed. Now I understand that I must receive some form of chemotherapy. Is it because the cancer has not been removed completely?"

"Your story is unfortunately not unique. As I already explained, it is indeed advisable for you to receive a six months course of chemotherapy not because some of the cancer was not removed but because even though it has been removed completely from where it was, its appearance and local extent when it was found were such that it is associated with a relatively high risk of recurrence in the form of metastases in the future (1). As I said before, in general the treatment of breast cancer in men is very much the same as in women."

I went on to explain to him in detail the reasons for which I recommended the treatment that would include chemotherapy and hormonal therapy, its potential benefits, limitations, side effects, risks and alternatives (2).

"While I have explained to you the reasons why I recommend that you receive that treatment, the decision about whether to go ahead with it is yours. You are the one to make it in the context of you own life style and priorities. Still, you must remember one thing and that is that the treatment can diminish the risk of appearance of metastases in the future or delay that event. While it may have its role in effecting a cure this is unfortunately not a guarantee that this will indeed happen. On the other hand, you may well already be totally free of any cancer although still at elevated *risk* of developing metastases."

He had just sat there listening to me explaining about the blood count, the nausea, the possibility of hair loss and all the rest of the tale of woes that goes with the chemotherapy (3), his mouth partly open, still incredulous about the whole thing.

"Boy! That is something to look forward to," he mumbled when I finished.

"The treatment is truly not that bad," I tried to reassure him. "I have painted the worst possible scenario for you just to tell you that these thing may happen, can happen, but do not necessarily happen and that even if they do they do not necessarily have to be bad. Most of these side effects are quite controllable to the point that your life will not be seriously disturbed. I explained to you the reasons for recommending it. Think about this for a few days, call me if you have any questions and if you decide to go on with my recommendations, we will get started."

He was quite calm as he got up from his chair but was shaking his head. "Of all the stupid things to have!" he mumbled. "I am quite sure I will go for the chemotherapy," he added, "but I still want to think for a couple of days if that is all right. Is it very urgent to start immediately?"

"No," I said, "but it is best to start soon. Call me by next week and let me know or make an appointment to start the treatment."

"Thanks Doc. See you soon, I'm afraid. Good bye".

Poor Fred. He did not know what hit him. He was still reacting to the first news of his cancer only now to face the fact that he had to receive chemotherapy, all that at time of his life when having worked hard and having accumulated a comfortable nest egg he should have been able to foresee an enjoyable retirement in the near future. It was not going to be that easy.

I see life as driving a car non-stop. If you drive long enough, something, a scratch, a fender bender, an accident, is bound to happen sooner or later. The longer you go the more likely it is to happen. Fred had been driving for a long time and the accident happened just as he was approaching home. Now the emphasis will have to be on repairs and preventive maintenance of the damaged vehicle of life. "Trade-ins for new ones not accepted," says the sign above the door of the repair shop.

Read chapters: (1) WHAT DID I DO WRONG?
            (2) DANDELION
            (3) WILL I LOSE MY HAIR?

WHAT DID I DO WRONG?

Chris was a young woman of twenty-nine, a slim, athletic and healthy looking brunette who had just been diagnosed with breast cancer. I had finished going over her history, had examined her and we were now sitting in my consultation room.

Her mother had died of breast cancer, as had her paternal grand mother. Needless to say Chris had understood early the reason for the repeated reminders to practice breast self-examination and she has done it. That is how she found that ugly-feeling tiny lump in her right breast. She had already gone through the surgery and the radiation therapy was planned for and scheduled to start. She was now coming to discuss other steps in her hopefully curative treatment. She was terribly disheartened at having developed breast cancer in spite of having maintained the lifestyle recommended for its prevention. "What did I do wrong?" she asked with tears filling her eyes. "I eat no fat, I keep my weight down, I exercise regularly, I neither smoke nor drink any alcohol or take any medications... and here I am with breast cancer. Did I neglect myself in any way? Am I being punished for something I have done? Why did this happen to me? What wrong did I do?"

She had come in my consultation room alone. Her father who had come with her had stayed in the waiting room at her request. He had come in to meet me only when they had just arrived and after the introductions he told me in a low voice which conveyed in a short sentence all the feeling of love I myself have for the one little girl in my family, "please take care of my little girl."

She was angry and frustrated.

It is shattering for any woman to have to face the diagnosis of breast cancer. But what about the physician who will take care of her? After forty years of treating women with breast cancer I still feel the stress when I have to answer these questions and even more so when then are, as they were on that day, asked by a woman young enough to be my daughter, who should be looking forward to a long and happy life, to sharing it with friends, to building and raising a family may be in the not too distant future, without worries about health...about death. Just thinking about it causes my heartburn to return and is the reason I still kept antacid tablets in my desk drawer.

"No you did nothing wrong. Women who have led a perfectly healthy life can develop breast cancer just as non-smokers can develop lung cancer. The reasons for this are still not completely clear but one thing is certain and that is that you must not blame yourself for your cancer. Neither are you being punished for any evil deed you think you may have perpetrated. The cancer just happened and now we both must look forward to try to cure it completely and permanently. What you did well however was to have remained on the lookout and that has paid off. You have found this cancer at a very early stage, at a time when it *can* be cured. You have taken good care of yourself."

"Can it really be cured? I thought that once you have had cancer that's it!"

"Not at all. That is not it at all! As a matter of fact, once its local treatment will be completed with the radiation therapy you may well consider yourself cured. Its size was fortunately very small and it has been removed entirely with a good margin of normal tissue around it. The lymph nodes that were removed from your armpit were found to be free of any cancer. This indicates that the cancer in all likelihood has not travelled beyond the breast. You will now go on with your course of radiation to the breast. Your blood tests, x-rays and scans show no evidence of cancer anywhere else, you feel well, you look well, and I find nothing abnormal on your physical examination. As far as I am concerned you have no detectable cancer."

"What should I do now?"

"Nothing other than periodic check-ups after you complete the radiation. The problem is that the absence of any abnormal findings does not always mean that there is definitely no cancer. It either means that indeed there is none or that, if there are any nests of cancer, they are so small that they cannot be detected by the available diagnostic methods. You are therefore still at a very small risk of having some microscopic clusters of cancerous cells surviving somewhere in your body. This probability is extremely small in your case but, because of it, I advise you to be checked at regular intervals from here on, more frequently at first and less frequently as time passes but at any time in between if any unusual symptoms develop."

"Should I receive any chemotherapy? I hear that nowadays every woman who has had surgery for breast cancer must receive chemotherapy."

"You hear right but you don't hear the whole story. Indeed, a significant proportion of women who have had surgery for breast cancer will relapse with the eventual appearance of breast cancer implants in other parts of the body even if no tumor tissue was found in the lymph nodes at the time of surgery. As you may know, these tumor implants are called metastases."

"Yes, I know."

"Among these women, however, some are at high risk of developing such metastases and those are the ones who should receive chemotherapy even if their lymph nodes were free of any cancer."

"How do you know which is which? I thought that the lymph nodes were the main factor, which would determine whether I would need chemotherapy or not and now you tell me otherwise. How come?"

I explained that lymph node involvement is one of the most important risk factors but not the only one. Other factors also have a role in determining this risk. The size of the initial breast tumor is another one with the probability of appearance of metastases increasing with the increasing size of this cancer. The microscopic appearance of the malignant tissue is yet another. This appearance varies: at one extreme the cancerous cells bear some resemblance to the normal breast tissue from which they have arisen and is described as moderately to well differentiated. At the other extreme, the cells are very bizarre-looking and are described as poorly differentiated. The former are generally the less aggressive ones and are associated with a better outlook while the latter are the more aggressive in spreading away from the breast and forming metastases and are associated with a relatively worse outlook. The finding of tumor cells inside blood vessels or lymphatic channels is likewise an indication of higher risk because such a finding indicates that these cells have penetrated the highways that may lead to other parts of the body. Simply measuring and examining under the microscope the tissue removed at surgery help in the evaluation of the aggressiveness of the cancer. They are the most important ones. Other tests conducted on the tumor tissue give some additional information in determining the outlook. One of them is the determination of the levels of the hormone receptors known as estrogen and progesterone receptors. This reflects the sensitivity of the cancerous tissue to alterations in the levels or presence of female hormones in the body fluids. Additional tests can reflect the rate of reproduction of the malignant cells while others determine presence of certain genetic markers associated with the potential course of the disease.

"Well, looking at all these where do you place me on the risk scale?" she asked.

This had been a lot of information to digest all at once but Chris was a smart young woman.

She wanted to know what she was up against and knew which questions to ask.

"You had a small cancer," I explained, "moderately well differentiated, without any invasion of blood vessels or lymphatic channels, with all lymph nodes free of cancer, estrogen receptor positive, progesterone receptor borderline and with other tests indicative of a low growth rate of the tumor cells. You are in the very low risk category for further spread of the cancer and need no additional treatment."

She took a deep breath and asked why not take chemotherapy anyway... for insurance.

"That," I explained, "is because not only is that treatment associated with possible toxic side effects but it is also not without some risk of potentially serious complications in the future. In your case this risk is at least equal to the risk of cancer while the benefit is quite small. Therefore one can truly say that it would not give you any worthwhile insurance while it may give you potentially serious unwarranted problems."

Most of the time, I have to convince the patient to accept chemotherapy as part of her initial treatment, yet on several occasions such as on that day I have had to convince someone of the fact that, because of her good prognosis, chemotherapy has nothing useful to offer her other than its inherent problems. The reason for this is the public's impression gathered from its erroneous interpretation of the media's reports, that *any* treatment carries with it some measure of effectiveness in every person afflicted with cancer. The truth is not only that many of the available forms of treatment are effective *only* against *some* of the cancers *some of the time* but also that the risks and side-effects associated with them may be such as not to warrant their use in low risk clinical settings.

"So what do I do now?"

"Now you make an appointment to see me again in about three months but remember that you may call at any time if you have any questions or problems. Take time daily to relax alone in the quietest place you may find. Give your mind a fifteen to twenty minutes vacation from all the problems of the day. Think beautiful thoughts while relaxing. Continue with your regular exercises. The exercise does not have to be exhausting. As a matter of fact it should not be. Yoga or Ta'i Chi may be the best because they give you relaxation along with poise and balance. Try it, you'll like it and you will feel much better. And yes, continue with your healthy diet. I don't know how preventive it is against the cancer but it is certainly good for your physical and mental well-being."

"Doctor," she said, still with tears in her eyes, "I will follow your advice. You have taken such a weight off my mind, off my soul! I already saw myself bald, sick and dying." She took a very long breath and started to cry. She sat in my office for a few minutes, then got up, squeezed my hands and gave me a kiss on the cheek. "Thank you she said" and left after wiping her tear-covered cheeks.

Yes, breast cancer is curable... frequently, although not all the time. It is certainly not hopeless. That conversation took place many years ago. Even then it had been known that certain families are plagued with a high incidence of several cancers among which breast cancer is prominent. The genetic determinants of this observation were not yet known but both Chris and I knew she was vulnerable. Breast cancer prevention was then a new concept without any concrete application. Periodic "check and see" were, and mostly still are, the major tools for early detection and for hope that treatment can be undertaken at a curable stage of the disease. Nowadays genetic testing and preventive measures are being actively investigated and have opened a door leading to more effective measures, in addition to early detection, in the fight against this disease.

WHERE THE ANSWERS?

One crystal ball slightly larger than a baseball contains clouds made of tiny air bubbles. The other, a little smaller, displays dark green shapes rising from the bottom and narrowing into points at about two third of its height giving the impression of a cluster of evergreens emerging from an icy island. For many years, I kept one or the other on my desk.

I have gazed into them often as a means of relaxing my mind for a few minutes between consultations or as a break from the accursed paper work that has become the plague of the medical practice and the nightmare of the medical practitioner.

These implements of the fortune-teller have served me in other capacities. They have been the equivalent of the "Nothing Device" that, many years ago, before the desk-top computers became so commonplace, had been featured in the catalogue of a very "pricey" department store. The "Nothing Device" was a clever gadget advertised for the man who already has everything. It consisted of a box that had all the outward appearance of a high-tech electronic device. It had a whole array of little lighted numbers, all arranged in neat high-tech looking rows, with all sorts of little control buttons that did absolutely nothing! These lights kept blinking in a totally random order. They blinked all the time. They never stopped for one instant. The particular characteristic of this clever gadget was that it could not be turned off other than by hitting it very hard with a sledge hammer or by waiting for it to die at the time of its programmed death, at which time it could not be resuscitated. The instructions that came with it clearly explained that peculiar characteristic of this esoteric piece of equipment. When that time arrived, it was described as "dead as a door nail." One of its listed potential applications was as a ploy to give to the high executive time to cogitate for a while about problems presented at board meetings without appearing to have any difficulty or to be at any loss for answers or solutions. He or she would get the box from behind the desk, place it on its top, punch a few of the useless buttons and gaze intensely at the blinking lit numbers as if looking for an answer to the problem of the hour. The big boss might even jot down some notes and looked tech-smart at a time when computer nerds did not yet exist. After this opportunity for reflection, "el jefe" could formulate appropriate and momentous decisions or comments. I don't think I could put up such an act without bursting out laughing after a minute. So, what did I do with my crystal balls? Very simply, when one asked me such questions as "What are my chances? Will this work for me? How long will I live?" and so many others to which I still have no answers, and provided I sensed that the person I was talking to was capable of accepting a truth laced with some humor, I would occasionally gaze into one of the crystal balls and shake my head in utter frustration. "This crystal ball is totally useless," I would finally say, "all I see here are green trees. Here, look for yourself," and I would hand it over. I would quickly add that such questions were normal but unanswerable. That acknowledgment of ignorance is still the most honest answer I can give to someone who then tells me that a friend who had been in the same predicament was "given" *x* number of months or years to live. Under such circumstances, even a little humor is accepted and it gives everyone a break from the seriousness of the circumstances. No one can "give" or state a limit to anyone else's life, particularly when options for effective treatment of an illness are still available and when the possibilities of new therapies are still wide open.

In recent years, I have had to store my crystal balls in one of the glass cabinets in my consultation room, all free space having been occupied by mounting sheaves of administrative paper to look at. Still, I prefer gazing through the clear substance of the crystal, and who knows, maybe one day I will see something in it. Until then, I have to continue doing it the hard way and limit my displays of wisdom to those few answers I really know.

NUMBERS

"Did you read the Sunday Times yesterday?"

That was in lieu of the usual greeting I got one day as I entered the examining room ready to check the next patient. I immediately knew what she was talking about.

"Yes," I answered.

"So did I. That was a truly frightening report about breast cancer. This is really scary!"

"I can certainly understand why and to tell you the truth I am very upset myself at the fact that such an article appeared in a newspaper."

"I gather from this article that I can expect to live about two and a half to three more years. That is not very much and it is very frightening... it is terrible!" She was almost hysterical.

"That is why I am very disturbed about it. Please try to calm down and tell me how you came to that conclusion?"

"It was there black on white! Considering the size of my cancer and the number of positive lymph nodes that you told me were found to be at the time of my surgery I fit in the group that will die in not too many years. I will not have the chance to get old. That is terrible!"

Joanne was truly shaken. I could see that she felt as if the rug had been pulled from under her. She was normally a high-strung person and now her world was crashing down around her. She was seeing her life as being over and all she had gone through had been for naught.

"Did you read that article carefully?" I asked her.

"Of course!" she protested. "It is all there in black and white."

"Then, like many people, you have missed something which is not emphasized in this type of article and which I will try to clarify for you.

20

The figure you quote as indicating the expected life span of someone like you is an *average* number." She wanted to say something but I motioned to her to listen for a moment. "Let me give you a simple example of one way of calculating this number: Let us assume that one study reports that over the last twenty years one thousand women presented the same findings as yours when they came to have surgery for their breast cancer. On review of their course over the years that followed some were found to have survived only three months, others survived six, still other lived one, two, four, ten or more years. Let us say that when the total number of months is calculated by adding all the survival periods it amounts to fifty three thousand months. Since there were one thousand women this figure is then divided by one thousand in order to determine the average survival per person. This comes to a fifty three months average survival. This is one of several ways of presenting statistical information but does that mean that you as an individual will live fifty three months?"

I stopped and waited for her to absorb what I had just said. She nodded signifying her understanding.

"Not at all. It means you may live three months, two years, ten years, or even that you may have no cancer left and that you may be cured. Completely and permanently cured. An average is an average. It applies to large numbers and not to individuals. It is used to evaluate treatment programs, compare them with others and plan further treatment strategies. It is not meant to tell people how long or how short a time they have left to live." I could see her starting to relax a little.

Furthermore, statistics, by their very nature, are based on information obtained in the past and does not necessarily apply to what will happen in the future since the field of cancer treatment is an ever changing and progressing one. No one knows what the future will bring.

"These figures are unfortunately quoted by the news media without appropriate interpretation or explanation. While informing the public is a very important function of these media, *that* information must be given in a form that can be clearly understood by those who will read it and in that and many other similar articles it is not the case. On the other hand, many such articles can also be very clear but are read selectively by the reader who retains only certain portions of the information and not others. The interpretation and the retention depend upon both the writer and the reader."

She was starting to regain her composure and took a few deep breaths.

"Thank you for making this clear to me," she finally said. "I am so relieved. Believe me when I tell you that I had already been planning my funeral, the obit, the announcements, the service, the meal, the drinks and, damn it, even the eulogy."

"Well don't. There is still a lot of good life in you. As far as I am concerned, you have no cancer and you are being followed only because of the risk. You have completed your chemotherapy and there is no sign of cancer anywhere. So go out and enjoy your life."

Now she gave me sad smile.

"I always try to but it is not easy. Wherever I turn and whatever news, I watch on TV or read in the papers the implication is that I am living on borrowed time. Numbers keep flying around me and it is awfully difficult for someone like me, without a medical background to interpret all this. Bad is always emphasized. I lay awake at night thinking about all this."

"If such thoughts creep into your mind at night," I advised her, "try this: think of a single beautiful and peaceful place where you may have been at one time or another, or visualize the most beautiful flower you can think of. Concentrate on that picture. Other thoughts may try to creep in but if they do banish them. Relax your body while doing this. It may be difficult at first but the more you do it the easiest it will become for you to relax both your body and your mind. You need this escape. You will even feel better in the morning and through the rest of the day if you do this successfully."

"No one can be protected from the assault of information you are talking about but one can develop a way to prevent it from being misinterpreted. Yet, while it is given correctly most of the time, it should be provided in the context of the information background of the reading public. It is frequently misinterpreted when read or viewed by observers with selective attention related to their particular problems. People select unconsciously some items and overlook others in the process of scanning the news. When they retain some of this information out of context it may become either unnecessarily frightening or falsely optimistic. If you want to read such an article in a newspaper or magazine," I added, "read it entirely, slowly and carefully at least twice before drawing any conclusions from it. Even then ask for translation into plain English and, make sure you call me before you start making any funeral arrangements, otherwise I will have to call the funeral parlor, cancel all their plans and mess up their schedule. They get very upset when this happens."

She left smiling.

Words, written or spoken, assume a life of their own, and a powerful one! Speeches have started revolutions. Edicts have resulted in murders, executions, or reprieves. Rumors have destroyed lives. I even recently read a book written by a well-known French lawyer titled "The Truth About Lies" in which the power of words, good or bad, is discussed in depth. Nowhere has the written word had as much power as when it applies to the survival or death of an individual. I constantly have to review newspaper clippings brought in or sent to me for comments about how or whether the information they provide applies to the treatment and survival of the person who brings it to my attention. The impact of this information is frequently so profound that I have made it a rule to read the material and always answer those who send it or bring it to me. Another rule is that I will *never, ever* state a limit to anyone's life.

WILL I LOSE MY HAIR?

Beth, the new patient of that day, was thirty-eight years old and yet looked like a young girl, slim with short wavy light brown hair. She had just embarked on the breast cancer journey and I was going to tell her of the potential dangers along the road and about the measures that could be implemented in order to minimize or prevent them. I had taken her medical history, examined her, and had reviewed all the records she had brought in. Now came the time for the summation of the findings and for the treatment recommendations. Two weeks previously she had undergone a lumpectomy for a cancer of the right breast along with removal of the lymph nodes in her armpit. Two of the nodes had been found to contain deposits of breast cancer and consequently I was about to advise her about the need for further treatment. This was going to be a two-hour session I usually reserve for a new breast cancer patient.

She had come with her husband and her mother. As they walked into my consultation room filled with piles of medical journals waiting to be "processed" (translation: discarded outright, perused briefly and then discarded or read and then kept and filed chronologically), one could feel the tension and anticipation of disturbing news.

My first words had to calm down the fear and anxiety that transpired through the calm but tense appearance of this family group.

"Before we go any further with this consultation," I started addressing the young woman, "I will tell you something which you must remember through the rest of today's conversation and beyond." All three looked at me somewhat puzzled. "Right now," I continued, "for all I or anyone knows, you may well be completely and permanently cured of your breast cancer!" I then waited a moment to allow the

24

impact of what I had said to sink in. Pursuing this train of thoughts I went on: "These are not idle words for there was a time not so long ago when all that was done for breast cancer was surgery. The breast used to be removed entirely along with all the lymph nodes. This was most of the time followed by radiation applied to the chest wall and local lymph node regions and that was all. No other treatment was given. In those times, nothing else would be done in terms of general treatment with chemotherapy unless the cancer showed, somewhere along the way, evidence that it had spread to other tissues in the body. Still, it was observed that many of the women who had gone through that type of treatment had no further problems for the rest of their lives and they were truly cured. The possibility and probability that you may be already cured are therefore real. On the other hand, many other women with the same disease and surgery were not so fortunate and over variable periods of time they showed evidence of spread of this same cancer to other parts of their body. At that time, they required additional treatment with medications in the form of chemotherapy or hormonal therapy. You are undergoing the same steps in the initial treatment process at this time except for the fact that instead of having had your entire breast removed along with the cancer only the cancer was removed by means of a wide excision leaving most of the breast intact. Now the remaining portion of the breast will be treated with radiation thus accomplishing by the fire, so to speak, what used to be done entirely with the knife."

I could see my listeners settling into their chairs but listening attentively. Because they were now anticipating an explanation of this process, curiosity and hope were slowly replacing the initial fear and anxiety.

"Two questions eventually came up: among those who had undergone surgery for breast cancer could we identify at the time of surgery those who were likely to relapse in the future with spread of the original cancer and should we wait for the proverbial other shoe to fall before initiating a treatment? Should we not instead try to prevent or at least delay the relapse in this group by applying treatment at the time of diagnosis rather than wait until the spread of the cancer becomes evident? As importantly, could we identify those at substantial risk of future relapse.

They were all listening.

"I am explaining all this to you in anticipation of all the questions I am sure you have and in order for you to understand the reason for the recommendations I will make at the end of this explanation. So listen carefully, try to hold your questions until I finish and then ask any that I may not have already anticipated during the course of this talk. You will have ample time to ask them. Feel free to interrupt me however if you do not understand something I say."

Over the years I had made it a rule to schedule new patients at the end of the day's work. The purpose was to give me the time to give them a comprehensive explanation of their problem and of its treatment and also in order to allow them time to ask all the questions they might have at that first session without having to watch the clock.

They settled back in their chairs now assured of the fact that I was not going to rush them in any way. From where they sat they could look at the bunch of colorful fancy Greek "worry beads" hanging on the wall by the door. Next to it hung a very simple framed pencil drawing of a mother and child titled "love," which had been executed by one of my patients who had given it to me several years previously.

"The reasons why some women are cured simply by the local treatment of breast cancer, whichever it is, and others are not has become better understood over the years," I continued. "Try to follow my explanation. It will not be technical: In order to be able to find a cancer in the breast it has first to grow to a size that makes it detectable or cause a symptom. One must be able to feel it with the fingers or it has to cast a characteristic shadow on an X-ray film. Size is therefore an important determining factor in its detection. It is impossible to detect a lump the size of a grain of rice or of an apple seed. Most of the cancerous lumps detected in the breast are at least the size of the tip of my small finger. I say at least because this depends also upon the size and the structure of the breast in which that lump develops. It is easier to find a small lump in a small soft breast but that lump may have to be three to four times larger before it is detected by finger palpation in a large lumpy breast. In general mammograms done routinely may detect even lesions which are frequently small enough to be non-palpable. Nevertheless, by the time such a tumor has reached the size that makes it detectable by any means it may already contain thousands or even millions of cancer cells. This growth process starts with a small cluster of a few cells and it takes time for it to grow from this limited cluster to the numbers of cells that make up the lump that is eventually detected. Based on our understanding of how long it takes for one cell to become two and two to become four, etc., as well as of the fact that the rate of growth varies, it is estimated that it may take that tumor months and possibly years to achieve the detectable size."

Addressing the young woman, I added, "In other words the cancer that was found in your breast although relatively small must have been there for a long time, undetected and *undetectable.* It appears to grow slowly for a long time and then suddenly, there it is. It is a little like compound interest at a rate of 100 percent. One dollar becomes two, two become four... one hundred become two hundred... one million become two million, and then suddenly the next time, while this sum grows at the same rate of interest, the number of units seems to go skyrocketing. That is when suddenly over a relatively short interval of time a lump that had not been found the last time you were examined is now present. It was there all along but could not be found even if you looked for it because it was too small."

She nodded as a sign of understanding.

"Now all this means is that there is a long period during the occult, non detectable, growth of this cancer during which it has ample opportunity from time to time to release some of its cells into the circulation via lymphatic channels or blood vessels. All are capable of doing that... all of them. Yet, some women are cured simply by the mechanical removal of the local cancerous tissue with or without the rest of the breast and the lymph nodes and, depending on the characteristics of the tumor, with or without radiation treatment to the remaining breast. So what happens to all the cells that were released in the circulation and that traveled throughout the body? Fortunately, the majority of these cells do not survive and if none survive and if all the local cancer and neighboring tissues have been removed by surgery the person is *cured.* On the other hand, some of these cells may survive in some patients and, if they do, they may plant themselves anywhere the blood or lymph stream has carried them to, which means anywhere except the hair, the nails and the teeth. These microscopic implants are so small that they are at first undetectable. Again, it takes them months and sometimes many years before they grow to a size that makes them manifest. That critical amount of cancerous tissue may have to be quite sizeable if it is hidden inside the body... and therein lies the problem.

How can we prevent or delay the growth of these microscopic tumor implants whose existence we suspect but we do not even know for sure?"

"Should we then treat every woman who has had a breast cancer operated upon with anti-breast cancer medications on the assumption that there are still malignant cells present in her body? The answer to this question would be unequivocally 'yes' if such treatment were either completely safe, without uncomfortable side effects and without any risks of its own, or if it were guaranteed to kill each and every residual breast cancer cell in the body. Unfortunately, all such treatments carry risks as well as uncomfortable side effects, nor are they guaranteed to result in a cure. What has been done, therefore, has been to try to identify risk categories for the breast cancer patients. We try to determine the relative likelihood that any one of them may develop evidence of spread of the cancer in the form of metastases in the future. If the risk is high enough to exceed the potential problems of the treatment itself, then an anti-cancer treatment is recommended."

I waited a moment for any questions but there were none.

"The risk is determined by the surgical findings, the pathological examination of the tissues removed at surgery (1) and of some special tests performed on the cancerous tissue itself." I explained the association of these morphological and biological findings with the magnitude of the risk of spread of the cancer. "If the evaluation of these factors is found to indicate a higher than minimal risk of eventual appearance of metastases then an anti-cancer treatment is recommended."

I stopped again for a moment. "Do you follow me so far?"

"Yes," answered Beth. "So, what happens now?"

"I will now go over the reports of your own tumor (1). In your case, the cancer was two centimeters in size and there were two lymph nodes invaded by breast cancer. Either one of these findings alone would indicate enough of a risk to recommend treatment with some anti-cancer treatment."

"Will I lose my hair? (2)" she asked moving forward on her chair.

"For heavens sake, don't be concerned about your hair," her husband interrupted, "we are here to talk about your health!"

Tears filled her eyes.

Of all the side effects of chemotherapy, I have found that the most disturbing is the hair loss associated with several of the anti-neoplastic medications. For the woman who has already suffered in her femininity through the loss or alteration of a breast and contemplating interference with her fertility, the emotional impact of the additional and very visible alteration in her appearance, if the therapy is of a type associated with hair loss, is shattering.

"This is a very understandable concern," I told them both. "Hair loss, for a woman, is undoubtedly an important consideration because it is so visible, and I will not minimize its impact. Yes, it is highly probable that you will lose hair but the severity of the loss may vary according to the treatment and to your own biology. Try to concentrate on the benefits of the treatment rather than that temporary hair loss in addition to your other problems, as difficult as it may be. I will explain it all to you as I put it in the context of the entire treatment."

She kept on dabbing her eyes with a tissue. Her husband held her hand as I continued.

"As I told you earlier, while you may well be completely and permanently cured of your cancer at this time, you do remain at significant risk of harboring some microscopic nests of breast cancer somewhere in your body. Because of this I recommend treating you as if this were indeed the case."

"I don't understand," she said.

"It means that I will *assume* the worst, that you truly have some cancer deposits present somewhere and treat you as I would if it were truly proven. I will recommend the same anti-cancer medications, the same dosage, the same frequency as given to people who have obvious progressive cancer but with one major difference. While in patients with proven spread of the cancer, a treatment of some sort is generally of lifetime duration on and off, in a situation in which the treatment is based only on the assumption of the presence of cancer the duration of that treatment is finite. It is given for a period of about five to six months at the end of which, if there is still no evidence of any cancer activity the treatment stops. There may be longer treatment with hormonal therapy to follow. Remember that you are treated only because of the risk, not because of the certainty of the presence of some cancer still tucked away some place in your body even after the breast surgery. The treatment stops therefore because, as I said earlier, you might not have any cancer deposits anywhere to start with. Then also, in the event that you had some microscopic deposits of cancer, the chemotherapy may well have done away with those and, in the absence of any concrete evidence of disease at the end of this period, one would not want to continue giving potent and toxic medications unnecessarily. Indeed, these medications are not without drawbacks in terms of their potential toxic side effects and risks. That is why their use in the absence of any demonstrable cancer after surgery is entirely based on the risk, the likelihood that undetectable cancer may still be present. Again, if that likelihood is very small the risk of the treatment itself may equal or surpass that of the cancer and it would therefore not be appropriate to recommend it. Once the risk of the cancer is high enough, treatment with chemotherapy becomes recommendable. Do you still follow me?"

They all nodded positively but the young woman had a question.

"If there is a possibility that I might not have any cancer left in my body, and, if as you just said, I may be cured now, why not wait, check me regularly and treat me if and as soon as the cancer does re-appear?"

This was a logical question and I told her that if she did not mind, I would address it as soon as I had given her all the information about the chemotherapy itself. "Chemotherapy may be administered in various combination of medications," I explained, "some of which can be given by mouth and some by intravenous injection. Those used in your situation have certain side effects in common and I will explain them to you. They affect mostly the cells that are growing actively such as cancer cells and that is good. Some normal tissues in the body also have an active rate of growth and are therefore also vulnerable to these medications. Those are the tissues where the toxic side effects of these anticancer chemicals will occur. These tissues are the bone marrow that constantly produces new blood cells, the hair follicles that constantly produce the growth of hair, the lining of the digestive system from the mouth to the anus because this lining is constantly active in the digestive process as well as shedding and replenishing itself, and the ovaries where eggs are maturing and being released each month in young women. Other tissues may also be affected to a greater or lesser degree."

I then proceeded to explain clearly and simply the major potential and occasional side effects and risks of the medications included in the chemotherapy regimen I was recommending: the nausea, the diarrhea, the fall in blood count, the possible hormonal changes, urinary symptoms, possible heart problems, nerve damage as well as effects on the skin and hair. I dwelt a little longer on some of them. I also told her about the relatively very small risk of leukemia associated with some of the chemotherapy medications.

"Ask me now or call me at any time if you have any questions about all this," I added before addressing her main concern. "While one or the combination of the medications I will recommend for you will produce a total hair loss this will be temporarily. Once the treatment is completed, the hair will start growing back and it will frequently be thicker, darker and curlier than before. Eventually, it will return to its previous texture and color. If you decide to go on with the chemotherapy, my advice will be for you to buy a wig that looks like your hair, as soon as possible. You will not start losing it right away and so you do have time. Your hair is short and the way it is set should be easy to match. You will realize that your appearance will not change once you have it on. If any of the side effects is severe and unmanageable the chemotherapy may have to be readjusted. Your periods may become irregular and may even stop but this does not necessarily mean that you will immediately be infertile. I will address this issue later."

I did not feel it was appropriate to discuss this issue with the patient and her husband in the presence of her mother.

"Since you are under the age of forty and even if your periods stop during the treatment, they are more likely to return within a few months after completion of the chemotherapy than if you were over the age of forty. Again, here I am talking about probability and not about certainty. One of the medications has an additional potential side effect that is to affect the cardiac muscle if a certain total cumulative dose is exceeded. Cardiac monitoring must be done periodically. This toxic dose to the heart will in all probability not be achieved in your setting and furthermore there are ways to minimize this potential problem. I will address this if and when the chemotherapy is agreed upon and its schedule is to be set."

"In a nutshell, some or all of these side effects may or may not occur and as I told you earlier, most of them may be easily controlled if not prevented altogether. Do not anticipate the worst. I have given you the information just so that you understand that if any of the symptoms occur it does not mean that anything is necessarily terribly serious."

"In addition to the possible side effects I have already mentioned that some risk may be also associated with the treatment. Fortunately, this is very small compared to the breast cancer risk that has warranted this chemotherapy in the first place. There may be any other unusual side effect, that may be the result of an individual sensitivity or idiosyncrasy to one of the medications. Therefore, if you receive the treatment and you experience some unusual symptom make sure you report it at once to the physician taking care of you or to one of us here should you decide to be treated in this office."

"I usually administer a pre-medication which will prevent most of the immediate side effects and I prescribe others to be taken at home to prevent those that may happen later. Believe me when I tell you that you will find the experience of your treatment here to be anticlimactic. There will be neither thunder nor lightning." She smiled. "Many of the people who come for their treatment at mid-day bring their lunch with them and eat it while the chemotherapy is going on. They frequently have a family member or a friend sit in the room to keep them company. They may read a book or sleep or listen to music or relaxation tapes on a portable tape recorder. In other words all of us here try to make that experience as little unpleasant as possible. You will find that although you are able to continue your usual day-to-day activities you may not have your usual stamina during the period of chemotherapy. Don't force yourself physically. Your energy will return within a few weeks after the treatment is completed. Try to maintain your usual lifestyle as close to normal as you can without strain."

"I have just given you all the bad news about chemotherapy but what *good* can it do for you? In women with the same clinical setting as yours it has decreased the risk of developing metastases although it has unfortunately not eliminated it completely. In other words it is not a sure cure. It means that in the appropriate and same risk category, women who have received chemotherapy have fared better than those who have not, in two ways. Cancer metastases have on the average appeared later in those treated than in those not treated and, during long periods of observation, there was a smaller number of women developing metastases among those previously treated than among the others. Unfortunately this also means that in spite of the treatment breast cancer can still reappear as metastatic deposits at any time and that more treatment will then be required. That is why even after the treatment is completed a program of regular follow up will be instituted.

Assuming I had finished my "exposé" the young woman asked: "What if I decide not to have any chemotherapy at this time?"

"I was coming to that but first I will answer the question you had asked earlier about why chemotherapy is recommended now instead of watching and waiting to see if indeed cancer starts growing again and treat at that time. The reason for treating now is that now if there is any cancer present it must be in the form of microscopic or very small deposits. Microscopic deposits of cancer are much more vulnerable to chemotherapy than larger ones. This has been established through experimental tumor studies as well as clinically. Therefore, if one wants to try to go for cure or best possible long term control the time to do it is now. If I may use an analogy, cancer is like a hungry tiger. If you come upon it when it is as small as a kitty-cat and your weapon is a heavy mallet, a heavy blow will most likely be able to kill it flat or to disable it for a very long time. If you come upon it when it is an adult, you may hit it with same mallet and stun it, cripple it temporarily, but you may find that it will soon get up and threaten you again each time although you hit it again and again. The same animal is more vulnerable at one stage of its development than at another. It is the same with cancer and although the mechanism of this is somewhat more complex, the analogy is still valid and that is why it best to treat now."

"A question you have not asked is why use several medications at the same time. The reason for this is that while I am talking to you about your cancer as breast cancer, all its cells do not behave exactly the same way biologically. They are all recognizable as breast cancer just as an animal of the dog family is recognized as canine. Yet, they do not all behave the same way. A wolf does not behave like an Irish setter neither can you control it the same way. A pack of diverse canines will require a combination of methods of control in order to tame it. If each breast cancer cell were exactly the same as any of the others all we would have to do would be to find the single drug which kills one of them and we could kill them all. Unfortunately, as I explained earlier they behave in several different ways and require several different medications simultaneously for best control and administered in a way that is also tolerable to the body which surrounds that cancer. Finally, I will answer your last question which is what would happen if you decided not to receive any chemotherapy at this time. I can simply put it that way: I have explained to you the fact that you are at higher than minimal risk of still harboring some microscopic breast cancer deposits somewhere in your body although there is also the possibility that you have none and that you may indeed be cured. I also explained to you that at this time the risk of the cancer is much greater than the risk and problems of the treatment. I have explained why it is best to treat now since now is when cure might be achieved if cancer is still present. Finally, I explained what you can expect from the treatment, what you cannot expect, its toxic side effects and its risks. I have also finally told you why I have recommended this particular treatment. It is now up to you to put all this in the context of your lifestyle and your priorities and to decide whether you wish to go ahead with it or not. You will be making this decision with as full an understanding of what you are up against and of what can be achieved. Now, if you are cured and receive no treatment nothing will happen. If you are not cured, meaning that there are some minute cancer deposits somewhere, these will eventually grow and are more likely to show up and show up earlier if no treatment is administered at his time. When they do, treatment will have to be given but the outlook will be more serious. I wish I could be more definite but all I can say is that if there is any possibility to move you from the 'not cured' to the 'cured' box the best time to try it is now. Whatever you decide that decision will be the right one for you. If I could have promised you a sure cure, you would not have to be convinced to receive the chemotherapy. It would be an automatic part of the treatment. You don't have to give your answer immediately. Give yourselves time to think for a couple of days if you wish and let me know your decision."

She was thoughtful for a little while. No one spoke for a couple of minutes and then she asked: "But if I start receiving the chemotherapy and I find out that I simply cannot take it and I want to stop it, how can I do that?"

"Very simply," I replied. "All you have to do is tell me that you want to stop and that will end this particular treatment. The fact that you started it is not a commitment for you to continue it. It can be stopped from one day to the next without any problem. We will then discuss the alternatives." Silence prevailed for a few seconds then her mother spoke: "I have a few questions although you have already answered many that I had thought of. May I go ahead now?"

"Of course. Now is the best time to ask all the questions you still have."

Read chapters: (1) WHAT DID I DO WRONG?
(2) THIS IS NEW YORK

ALL THESE MEDICATIONS

"What will all these medication do to her immunity?" her mother asked. "Does it not weaken it and is it not bad for the person with cancer to weaken the immunity?"

Beth's mother was looking at a small notebook on which she had apparently written some questions. She had already drawn lines across a number of them that I had already anticipated and answered during our earlier conversation. She had told me that she was a retired Nurse.

"Theoretically, you are right, anti-cancer medications do cause some suppression of immunity. Yet, in spite of this, the reality is that women have fared better with treatment than without it. These are the observed facts. Some cancers have even been cured by intensive chemotherapy. What else can I tell you other than that is the proof of the pudding? Besides, what good was her immunity doing while the cancer was growing?"

"What about diet? How can she strengthen her immune system?"

"I wish there were something as easy as a diet to strengthen the components of the immune system that would specifically attack breast cancer or any other cancer for that matter. The truth of the matter is that very little is known at present about which, if any, nutritional elements or supplements are capable of offsetting the immunosuppressive effects of chemotherapy. It is known that there are lifestyle and *nutritional lifetime habits* that are associated with a lower incidence of breast cancer in certain populations but there is not enough evidence to support that a change to such a dietary program can be effective in altering the course of an already established cancer. I can give you the names of physicians who make a study of the role of nutrition, vitamins and other supplements on cancer and on the immune system and you may wish to consult one of them for any useful recommendations and dietary regimen. All I can advise in terms of diet at this time is to follow what may be best called the 'prudent diet.' This means mainly cutting down the consumption of animal source fat such as found in red meat, whole milk products, butter, cream, margarine, prepared desserts, ice cream and the like. It means cooking with little fat and eating no fried foods or cured meats. Some vegetable oil is OK. Fish is a good source of protein, poultry is not bad as long as it is skinned and all the fat removed before it is cooked, white meat being better than dark parts, and limited amounts of well trimmed and well cooked red meat. Vegetables are fine. Try to cook them without fat or with a little oil. Desserts...Ah yes, desserts! ...God did not put apple pie and ice cream for us as dessert. God has given us fresh fruits of all types for that purpose. That is the best dessert you can have. Fruit is sweet, it changes the taste after a meal, it is refreshing and generally lower in calories than the prepared desserts and finally has no fat. Yes, fruit for dessert. One more thing: calories. Do not overeat because for some reasons, some clear and some unclear, people tend to gain weight on chemotherapy. Try to keep your weight stable."

Her face told me some thing was not clear to her.

"I thought people lost weight with chemotherapy," Beth interjected. "I thought they got sick and could not eat."

"Not so," I replied. "Actually most tend to gain. It may be because they eat the same amount of food but are less active, or because they feel a little nausea and find that if they nibble on something it relieves it and therefore they eat more. Others believe that weight loss is a sure sign of progression of the cancer and they try to eat more and gain weight as reassurance that the cancer is not progressing. Finally, there may well be some change in metabolism that may be related in part to the disturbed function of the ovaries and in part to mechanisms that are not clear but that result in weight gain. So watch yourself. Weight gain is not necessarily healthy. Don't try to lose but try not to gain any either."

"The importance of diet for the prevention of metastases in people who already have a diagnosis of cancer is not at all established. While there are epidemiological studies linking diet and lifestyle to the *risk* of developing breast cancer, there are no good studies to date that have linked the risk of metastases to such diets *after* the cancer has already appeared. It is more likely that *life-long* dietary habits influence the incidence of certain cancers in some parts of the world. All I can tell you about the diet I have just explained to you is only that it is healthier than the average American diet as we know it and I recommend it on that basis."

"What about vitamins?" she asked.

"There is some experimental evidence that certain vitamins such as vitamin C, vitamin E, and beta carotene and may be some of the trace elements in the diet, have some general anti-cancerous properties but it is again not clear whether starting to take these after the genesis of a cancer will affect its ultimate course over and above what the chemotherapy can do. I see no harm in taking a supplement in the form of a daily multivitamin tablet. If you want to explore diet as an adjunct to the chemotherapy, I can look for and refer you to a group that is doing this on an investigational basis. This means the investigators are trying to find out what diet and vitamins do by comparing those on a regular regimen with those on a program of special diet and various supplements such as vitamins, etc."

"I don't think I want to get into any study program at this time," said Beth. "Are there things I must avoid?"

"None other than what I already mentioned as well as any medications containing estrogenic (female) hormones. Since they have a role in stimulating or maintaining the growth of breast cancer, they are best avoided. This may well apply also to food items containing a significant amount of the so-called natural plant estrogens."

She gave a long sigh.

"I think I will go ahead with the chemotherapy although I do want to have a chance to think about it for a couple of days as you suggested, and digest what you said. If I do start can you take care of it here in your office?"

"Of course. This is what we do here, and by the way, while you were in the waiting room filling your questionnaire, did you see a number of patients come in and out of the office?"

"Yes."

"Did you notice anyone to appear particularly ill?"

"No."

"Yet, at least half of them had just received their chemotherapy here. So as you already noticed it is not anything as horrible as frequently depicted in the magazines and other news media."

"Should someone accompany her when she goes for chemotherapy?" asked her mother.

"It may be a good idea to have someone come along the first couple of times until I see how she manages. If she feels all right, she may come by herself thereafter. Many people do that on their own. It is truly a matter of the individual person's reaction to the medications, not that she will feel terribly ill but she may feel tired, and the presence of someone with her may make her feel more comfortable. We can play that by ear."

"May I continue to work asked Beth or should I tell my boss that I need time off for my treatment?"

"It is truly up to you. My usual recommendation is to try and see if you feel well enough to maintain your job. If you can, I feel you are better off continuing to work. It keeps you busy, keeps your thoughts off the subject of your cancer and your treatment, not counting the economic advantage."

"That sounds right. I still have a few days off and may try and see how I fare with the first treatment. I can always decide later."

She thought for a moment and then "I have one more question," she said. "How will you know if the treatment is working?"

"I will not know if it is working but I will know if it is not," I replied watching the amazed look on their faces. "There is no way I can find out if it is working because there is nothing to follow, nothing to measure. You have no detectable cancer, nothing I can see become smaller or disappear. I am not treating a concrete entity but only a risk. On the other hand, if the cancer reappears somewhere while I am treating you or shortly after the treatment has been completed it will be proof that the treatment was not effective. That is why some follow up is recommended not only during the treatment but even after the treatment has been completed, more frequently initially and at longer and increasing intervals as time goes on."

"But," she retorted, "if you cannot tell what happens, of what help is the follow-up since there is nothing to follow?" I then explained to all three what information the follow up visits would provide: "When I see you at your follow-up visit I start by asking you how you feel and if anything unusual has happened to you since the previous time. Then I also examine you. My eyes, hands and ears being also limited in their capacity to detect very early signs of cancer activity I request periodic blood tests that may reflect the function of different organs in your body and that may give me additional information about your state of health. It is also necessary from time to time to obtain imaging studies of those body portions or organs most vulnerable to the spread of that cancer. I then put together all the information obtained by your responses, my examination and the results of the tests and I evaluate the combination of what comes out. Assuming that all results are normal I can only conclude that, to the best of my ability to look for evidence of cancer activity, I can find none with the means available to me. It may mean that either there is no cancer at all or that, if there is any, it is to small or of too limited activity to be detectable it by available methods. If any abnormality is disclosed in the course of that evaluation, I then follow it in order to determine if this is the result of some unrelated illness, an effect of the treatment of if it is related to the cancer itself."

"So if I go five years without any problems, will I be home free?" she asked again.

"In the past, five years without clinical recurrence of the cancer was considered to be the limit after which it could be considered to be cured. This concept has changed. Indeed, most of the metastases, if present, will manifest themselves within the first five years and even within these five years the first two make up the period of the greatest frequency of these recurrences. Still, it has been observed that metastases could and did occur during the following five years although much fewer in numbers. And so one started to talk more in terms of five or ten years *disease-free* period rather than *cures* although a ten year disease free survival is most frequently equivalent to a cure. Unfortunately, we have all seen metastases appear occasionally even after ten years. I have seen it very rarely even after twenty years but beyond that it almost never happens."

She was teary again. "Are you telling me that I will never be cured?" she asked.

"Not at all. I will again repeat what I tried to convey to you earlier: you may be cured right now. You may well be totally free of any cancer already. What I am saying is that some women may not be cured at the stage at which you are now and that in these particular women the cancer may manifest itself again sooner, later or very much later. No one can tell at this time who is going to do what and that is unfortunately the nature of the beast that is breast cancer. What I can tell you is that the longer you go without any evidence of metastases the longer you are likely to go. What I can also tell you is that those women whose cancer reappears many years after the diagnosis is established at the time of breast surgery, are those who tend to respond best and longest to further treatment and who are likely to go on with long and comfortable survival even with metastases. At this point let us accentuate the positive, like in the song, and plan that all will go well. It is the best way to look at the future. Stack the deck in your favor and hope for the best."

"Do you really think I may be cured?" she almost implored.

"I think it is very likely."

There was a moment of silence then Beth turned to her mother: "Mom if you have no more questions we would like to talk alone for a few minutes."

"Of course" her mother said. She thanked and went out to the waiting room.

WHAT ABOUT SEX?

When she was gone, Beth turned first to her husband and then to me:

"What about sex?" she asked. "May we continue as usual? Can it be harmful?"

I noted once more in my mind that it is frequently the patient herself and not her husband who asks this question.

"Not at all. If your surgery does not cause you any discomfort there is no reason not to maintain your sexual relations as you would normally. Remember that the main reason for the treatment is to maintain your life as normal as can be achieved in spite of the temporary disruption. Sex is one of the good things in life and there is no reason to make any changes. I must warn you, however, as I said previously that if your periods become irregular or stop that does not necessarily mean that you are not fertile. I presume you have been using some method of birth control."

"I have been on the pill since we had our last child but I have stopped now. I have recently used a diaphragm."

"Fine. You should certainly not become pregnant while you are receiving chemotherapy. You should therefore continue to use whatever barrier contraceptive you are more comfortable with rather than birth control pills as you had in the past. This means using either a condom or a diaphragm and jelly. It may not be as practical as the pills but as I explained to you before it is best to avoid the use of any estrogenic medications for the present time."

"This should not be a problem," her husband added. "We already have our family of three children and have not planned to have any more."

"You may also find," I added, "that if your periods stop during chemotherapy you may develop some hot flashes as if you are going through menopause. That is most often a nuisance rather than a problem. The problem sometimes is the vaginal dryness that may be associated with it. If it is bad or causes discomfort at intercourse a vaginal cream such as KY Jelly or any other similar product applied before intercourse may frequently be all that is needed to manage this. If you have such a problem, talk to your gynecologist or talk to me. This is best and most easily resolved early if it happens at all. Try to maintain your normal sexual habits since it may be the best way to avoid any such difficulties."

They looked at each other to see if any one had any other questions.

"I guess we cannot think of any other questions right now," he said.

"You were very helpful she added. I am glad my surgeon referred us to you. He said you would explain it all to us and you certainly did. If I have any other questions, may I call you? I really cannot think of any but just in case."

"Of course."

"I am sure I will opt for chemotherapy but I need the time to think and I will let you know soon. This is a lot to digest."

"You will be surprised about how quickly the time will pass. It will look at first like this treatment will never end but it will before you know it."

"I hope so."

After they left and after so many similar conversations I ask myself if truth can really be made reassuring when it can be expressed only as speculations without definite knowledge of the facts. I guess it depends on the perception of the person at the receiving end, a perception filtered through her or his own fears, wishes and hopes.

RECONSTRUCTION

Damage sustained along the breast cancer journey may be small or large, serious or minor. It may or may not require repair. A decision about the latter rests mostly with the patient herself. Can life continue happily without repair of the surgical damage? Eleanor raised that question one day.

"Should I have breast reconstruction?" she asked as I sat at the examining room desk.

Eleanor was in her late fifties, a widow for seven years, with a full figure somewhat on the fuller size of that time's anorexic fashion. She had undergone a right mastectomy six years previously, wore an external prosthesis and looked great dressed. It was impossible to tell she had undergone major breast surgery except for the fact that she always wore dresses or blouses with a high neckline, even in summer, or turtle neck garments in winter.

We were still in the examining room with its wall decorated with pictures of flowers I had taken with my old camera and had enlarged and framed to add color to the rooms of my "establishment." Her regular examination was completed. She was still sitting on the examining table. Her bra containing the heavy silicone prosthesis had been placed on the chair beside it. The chest asymmetry was obvious even through the loose fitting salmon pink paper gown.

"Why now?" I asked.

"Oh, I have been thinking about it for a very long time," she replied, "actually ever since I had the surgery. With the chemotherapy, the five years of hormonal therapy, my husband having died, I put it all on a back burner. Now I started to think about myself. What do you think? Should I do it?"

"You are asking the wrong question. You ask me if you *should* do it and the answer to this is no because it is not a medically necessary operation," I explained. "The question should be whether there is any reason why you *should not* do it. My answer to that is also no. In other words, if it is important to you as a person to have your breast reconstructed there is no reason why you should not."

"Well I don't know," she said. "I am still hesitating. It is after all another operation and for a long time, although I wanted to have it done I kept asking myself what did I need more surgery for. Thank God and thanks to you I am doing well six years later. I passed the five year mark and now I feel the reconstruction will be a kind of reward for myself, a way of putting the final period to that part of my life and pushing it all behind me. What do you think?"

"Why don't you get dressed and let us talk about this a little more in my office," I suggested.

A few minutes later, she walked in my consultation room. She was tall, beautiful and elegant. As she sat, I asked her:

"In the examining room, were you truly asking my opinion about breast reconstruction or were you simply in your own way telling me you had decided to have it done?"

"I truly wish for your advice. As I told you, I am still hesitating. I feel very well. Am I not opening a Pandora's Box by having more surgery now? I am very ambivalent about the whole thing. I don't know what to do."

"Is it that you are unhappy about your self-image? If it is constant emotional burden for you to have lost a breast and if your physical appearance is a constant reminder of the fact that you have had cancer, then by all means start looking into reconstruction. If you are still unsure as to why you want to do this, you may give yourself time to reflect on it before you take that step. In the interim, get one or two consultations with plastic surgeons so that you understand how this is done and what type of result you may expect from the surgery. I will give you the name of an excellent one who will explain it all to you."

She hesitated a little.

"How can I put this?" she then added. She stopped for a moment, looking at her knees, as if to gather her thoughts or decide whether to continue. I waited. "There is more to it than my self-image and all that," she finally added, raising her head. "I lost my husband seven years ago and I then developed breast cancer within a year of his death and went through the surgery and the chemotherapy. I am now starting to live again." She stopped again for a few seconds and then continued as if in one breath. "A year ago," she recounted, "I met a man I liked very much. He is a professional man, also a widower, and we truly enjoyed one another's company. As our relationship grew closer, I began to dread the possibility of becoming more intimate with him in spite of my desire for it. How would he react to my mastectomy? I had not told him anything about it, which, now I know, had been a mistake, but I did not know how to tell him. I kept procrastinating. I eventually stopped going out with him and we drifted apart. Now I stay aloof of such relationships although I miss terribly the companionship of a compatible man. I have long thought about it during the past several months and I feel that, in many ways, I will be more at ease with myself if I have a breast reconstruction. I also realize that I must get the mastectomy story out in the open early in the course of any relationship, before it has time to develop into anything more serious or, having reached that point, cause it to sour as a result of its late discovery." She stopped again. "Now you may understand more about my reasons for considering this surgery at this time. I am ready for it in my head but still fearful of it physically."

"I think you have already answered all your questions yourself," I told her, "I understand why you are looking into it. This is a very individual decision. You have obviously thought it out but have not been able to take the last preparatory step that is to consult the plastic surgeon. Bear in mind that this will not solve all your emotional needs. If anything, it may be only a step toward facing the life ahead."

She remained silent for a moment.

"I understand that. I have thought a lot about it but did not have anyone to talk to. Only a few of my closest friends know I have had a mastectomy but I am not that close to anyone with whom I can discuss all this. I feel talking with you today has helped a lot." She decided to take my suggestion and seek a plastic surgeon's evaluation and information about breast reconstruction.

Four or five months later, Eleanor returned to my office for her follow up examination having undergone the type of surgery which uses an abdominal muscle flap to reconstruct the missing breast, and a little lift of the remaining one for symmetry. The result was excellent all the way to the nipple and areola, that had also been reconstructed along with the breast and tattooed for the right pigmentation. She was so happy she could now dress like any other woman. So there were scars but she no longer had to contend with special undergarments, a breast prosthesis which could shift in position, special bathing suits, and a limited dressing fashion. She told me about her feeling of freedom. She was now able to talk more openly about her experience with breast cancer, her mastectomy and her breast reconstruction. She expressed the fact that she had become more at ease socially. She had not found her soul mate yet but she no longer had the feeling of isolation she had expressed at the time of her previous visit.

"This is the renewed me," she told me that day. "It is not all the result of the reconstruction but mostly of the fact that I finally decided that it was time I stopped mourning the loss of that part of my body and get on with the life I wish to have and enjoy. I feel great and I thank you for helping me get on the right track."

I PAID MY DUES

...But repairs are not always essential for life to go on.

Joy had just completed her six months of chemotherapy after her mastectomy. When she had first come to see me, she had obviously been shattered by all that had recently happened to her after the discovery of a suspicious shadow of the mammogram of her left breast. It was first the needle biopsy, then the mastectomy followed by the news that she needed 6 months of chemotherapy. She had planned at the time to undergo breast reconstruction as soon as the chemotherapy would be completed. She could not stand the sight of her mastectomy and had confided to me the fact that she never looked at herself in a mirror until she had a garment on to cover that scar. She had frequently stated that she was anxious to finish with the chemotherapy in order to have her breast reconstructed. In the course of the recent months of treatment and examinations in our office she had become less uncomfortable with the fact she was missing her left breast and could now let me examine her mastectomy area without grimacing.

On that last day of chemotherapy, I asked her:

"So, are you making plans for the breast reconstruction?"

"I don't know," she replied. "At first, I could not wait to finish the treatment in order to go ahead with it. Now I am no longer sure I want to undergo more surgery. What do you think?"

"From what you are telling me I think you are obviously not ready for it although it seemed very important to you when you first came here. What happened?"

"As in the song, I got accustomed to my...shape with one breast. My husband loves me better than ever. I finished with the chemotherapy.

47

I feel that as of now I have paid my dues. I am not sure I am ready to put myself again through another surgery. I can always change my mind later can't I?" she asked.

"Of course. This is not an urgent procedure, neither is it a medically necessary one. You have all the time in the world to decide about it and you may change your mind. This is something that has to do with your self-image. If you find that you can live quite comfortably emotionally with yourself, you need do nothing else."

She smiled. "I think I will continue to live with that old battle-scarred body of mine and leave it as it is. I will consider that silicone breast in my bra as my medal for bravery under fire."

HE LEFT ME

Some will abandon ship at the initial forecast of the storm moving its way and such is the story of Gerry.

One day, several years ago, I received a letter from a physician located in Vancouver requesting information about a young woman I had treated over twenty years earlier. He was taking care of her younger sister and he was asking for details about the type of breast cancer my patient had had and about her clinical course, in order to evaluate that sister's breast cancer risk category. While I looked up the information, I recalled immediately the circumstances of this unfortunate young woman. I remembered her because she had been quite young at the time, while breast cancer has always been a disease most prevalent in women in their forties and fifties.

Gerry was thirty-two when she first consulted me, a slim, lively young woman, well informed about her illness and quite articulate. She had undergone a mastectomy for what was found to be an aggressive type of breast cancer. The initial consultation had been easy to complete. Both she and her husband had been in to see me together. She had answered most of the questions herself. It was soon obvious to me that he had been there mainly for moral support having said very little during the course of the interview and of the discussion of the chemotherapy program I had recommended.

Within a few days chemotherapy was started and, four weeks later, she was once again in my consultation room after her first follow up examination. I asked if her husband who I thought was in the waiting room was going to join us.

"Oh no! He is not here. He left me," she said.

Assuming he had to leave because it had taken so long to finish with the examination and the chemotherapy I apologized for the delay and told her he could call me if he has any questions.

"No, you don't understand," she said. "He really, truly left me" she repeated. "He is gone. He came only for the first consultation last month because I asked him to, but he had left me a week after my mastectomy."

This revelation had been uttered as simply and clearly as the rest of the information she had previously given to me. While I was surprised for a moment, this statement did not produce the element of shock it should have. Sadly Gerry's was not a unique case. I have treated a number of women of all ages who have had the same unfortunate experience complicating a life already undeservedly punished by the diagnosis and treatment of breast cancer. She sat there with her serious freckled face of a prematurely wise little girl framed by her short and curly red hair. I can still picture her in my mind.

"Did you have any indication that this was about to happen before your surgery? Were there any problems already existing between you and your husband?"

"No nothing unusual. We have had our disagreements over the years but when it happened it truly hit me like a ton of bricks. One morning exactly one week after I returned from the hospital he announced that he was leaving. He said he could not deal with illness. He just packed up and left...just like that. I didn't know what had happened. I was stunned."

"Have you thought about consulting a marriage counselor?"

"Yes I did, but he would not have any part of it. He told me in so many words that he wanted out. There was no arguing with him."

"So what happens to you now?"

"Now I have to take care of myself. I have the apartment. I am working and hope to continue. After that I don't know. I may go back to my family. We will have to go through the divorce. My husband is rather immature. I am certain he does not know what to do either but at this point that is his problem. I have an attorney who will help me. I have talked to her. She is a childhood friend and has been very supportive. I must get on with my treatment, my health, my life... as it is."

With her last statement she gave a sad smile with tears in her eyes.

"Indeed, you must get on with your life. Let us move on with your treatment for now. At least that is all planned and under way. We, you and I, shall accentuate the positive and get you over it during the next 12 months (at the time of this episode adjuvant chemotherapy was given over that period of time. This has changed since then). Still, I have one good piece of advice to give you. If you are close to your family stay close because in the final evaluation no one will give you the emotional and physical support you need as well as a close family."

As it turned out this unfortunate young woman had a very virulent cancer that progressed while she was undergoing the initial treatment. Eventually, she was treated under an investigative chemotherapy program that also failed to control the relentless spread of this malignancy and she died a few months later.

I always wondered about the influence of such personal unhappiness on the eventual outcome of the treatment of cancer. My personal observations that, while numerous remain anecdotal, have led me to think that women with good emotional and family support, particularly from a spouse, seem to fare better at least in terms of coping with the problems of the cancer and of its treatment. Whether this play a role in the actual response to treatment and in the survival is very hard to determine. I would not be surprised if one day we will find that it does.

A VOICE ON THE TELEPHONE

This episode occurred more than thirty years ago. In retrospect, it turned out to be a forerunner of questions that have been raised with the relatively recent discovery that genetic abnormalities of the BRCA-1 and BRCA-2 genes related to familial breast cancer. This was not known at that time. The main question was the one that asks what is a young woman to do in order to prevent breast cancer when she knows that her risk of developing it is many times higher that it is for the general female population.

A close friend told me about a young woman who was very concerned about her risk of breast cancer because of the large number of her female relatives who had suffered with it. She wanted to protect herself but did not know what to do or whom to call for advice. She had some foreknowledge of the danger of the breast cancer voyage and wanted to avoid embarking on it. Our friend told me she had taken the liberty to tell her to call me and discuss it with me. She thought I would not mind, and I did not. In preparation for this call I searched through the Index Medicus, that large series of volumes in which all medical publications were listed and classified over the years, for information about familial breast cancer. Before the era of computer databases, that tedious and long search through the heavy volumes of the Index was the only way to find the titles and location in the medical journals, of published medical articles on any subject. I searched for the titles of reports about families with a high incidence of breast cancer. Having found several I then went to the medical library of the Cornell University Medical College and pulled out the old bound volumes of the medical journals in which these articles had been published. What I found was that there were indeed families in which a major proportion of the women had developed breast cancer and those who had not developed it at the time of the report were considered to be at very high risk of developing this malignant illness in their lifetime. These families were rare and it was postulated that some genetic defect was the probable cause of this particularly high risk. That was as much as I could find on the subject at the time but it was enough to document the understandable concern of this young person.

A few days later she finally called me. She introduced herself at told me that our friend had referred her and did I know about her problem. I told her that I had expected her call. She just wanted some advice, did not really want to come to my office but would explain her predicament to me on the telephone. She then went on to tell me that of her five maternal aunts four had developed breast cancer and three of them had died of it as had her maternal grand mother. The only aunt who did not develop that cancer had convinced her physician to perform a bilateral mastectomy in the absence of any detectable breast problem. Then six months prior to that conversation over the wires her mother underwent surgery for breast cancer. The irony of this was that she had discussed prophylactic mastectomy with her physician citing her only healthy sister as an argument for this radical approach. He dissuaded her from it arguing that he was following her at close intervals with both mammograms and physical examinations of her breasts and that surgery could be done very early should she ever develop any suspicious lesion or mammographic change. When this finally happened, she was found at surgery to have an advanced stage tumor with metastases in multiple lymph nodes of the axilla. To top it all one of the young woman's first cousins, daughter of one of her dead aunts, a young woman of thirty-two, had undergone breast cancer surgery two weeks prior to her call.

Her question was: what should she do if anything as a single woman of thirty? All that on the telephone! She did not want to be examined. I could not even look at her to gauge the level of her anxiety, to guide me on how to talk to her. I first related to her the findings of my medical literature search. I then explained to her my conclusion that, based on her family history, indicated that she belonged to one of these rare families with a genetically transmitted high risk of developing breast cancer in her lifetime. While she could try to control some of the environmental and lifestyle factors that could be associated with an increased risk of this cancer, their role was very likely to be a very minor one compared to the role of the genetic abnormality. In the final evaluation, the choice was either that of close surveillance and acting only when a breast lump or an abnormal mammogram appeared, living with a sword hanging over her head, or of being pro-active and opting for a prophylactic bilateral mastectomy which under the circumstances was not very far-fetched and was a quite defensible option. At that time the surgical techniques of breast reconstruction were already quite good. This young woman had obviously given all of this a lot of thought already because none of what I said appeared to surprise or to upset her. I offered again to have her come to my office and discuss all this face to face after she had time to think about it and she thanked me for the offer which she would take advantage of if she needed it. She felt our talk had been very helpful to her and again thanked me. And that is where that conversation ended.

Eight to ten months later I received a call at my office from that same young woman.

"Remember me?" she asked after reminding me of our previous discussion.

"Of course! Tell me what has happened to you, what have you done?" I asked.

"You helped me make up my own mind. I had almost come to a decision before talking to you," she added, "but I needed to talk to someone like you and Bea was right in telling me to call you. Shortly after we talked I had a bilateral mastectomy and an immediate reconstruction, and I cannot tell you how relieved and happy I am to have made up my mind and to have had the surgery. I just thought since you had kindly taken the time to talk to me without even knowing me, that I ought to let you know the outcome of my quandary and to thank you again."

I wished her good health, long life and happiness. I hope she remains well to this day.

This young woman had witnessed her close relatives' voyage through breast cancer and had foreseen the possibility of going through it herself, a possibility she had wanted to avoid. She consulted, studied and planned for a different scenario and after due consideration she deliberately implemented it.

Bilateral mastectomy for the purpose of reducing or eliminating the risk of breast cancer is an option that, while drastic has been investigated and has been found to be effective. It still remains a difficult option to consider for the small proportion of women who are in this unusual high-risk group. Alternatives to this, in the form of medications, lifestyle modifications, or other non-surgical interventions, have been under very active investigation since discovery of the association of abnormalities of the BRCA-1 and-2 with a high incidence of cancer of the breast and of the ovaries. Prophylactic surgery including the removal of the ovaries as well as other preventive measures are still being explored.

THE PHOTOGRAPH

We all have within ourselves a small touch of paranoia. The stress of illness may accentuate it in some.

"Why the photograph?" she asked. "Is it for the before and after record?"

"No, it is just to place your picture in your medical record."

"That is interesting. I have never heard of it being done."

"I have been doing it for years. I just saw you for the first time today and you may eventually have your treatment here or you may go elsewhere and come only for follow up at long intervals. Or you may call me on a busy day. But whenever that happens and when I open that record I want to be able to see you and think of you as Jenny Woods and not as the right breast tumor on XYZ chemotherapy. I want to see you in my mind as a person, not as a disease. The picture helps."

"All right," she said, as she stood her back to the wall, "do I smile?"

"Sure you do, and with your smile you'll win the photo contest."

We both chuckled, the portrait picture was taken with my Polaroid camera, was taped inside the back of the chart and I waited in my office while she was getting dressed. Most patients truly appreciated the fact that I was doing all I could to consider them as real people and not as body carrying an illness to be treated. They were all grateful for that little touch that made them feel that when they came to be examined I cared for each one as an individual person. I think I was one of the first physicians to enter a photograph of patients in their record for that purpose. The more recent Polaroid device was much less cumbersome than the original model and was perfect for that purpose.

The only person who, after her only visit to my office, requested in writing to have her picture removed from the record and mailed back to her was a Chicago attorney. Who knows what nefarious ulterior plans she had attributed to my reasons, as she perceived them in her litigating lawyer's mind, for taking her picture and for inserting it in her record, other than the one I had stated.

I promptly mailed the photograph.

TO SHARE OR NOT TO SHARE

Sometime in the early sixties, at the hospital where I worked, a fund was created in memory of one of my deceased patients. Her friends and family had contributed to it after her death and it served to create and maintain for a couple of years, a group discussion about breast cancer. All the participants were women who had breast cancer at various stages of the disease from potentially cured to extensively disseminated and all of them were undergoing some form of chemotherapy. They were ten or twelve in all and all of them except one were under my care at the time although the group was open to breast cancer patients referred by any other physician and attendance was free. The novel idea at the time was to have the patients who had been or were currently treated for breast cancer converse openly with their physician about the problems facing them. There were no holds barred. We talked about the surgery that, at the time, meant radical mastectomy and its physical aftermath; its effect of their self image of femininity; the fear of cancer recurrence and of the chemotherapy treatment which would follow; the toll on relationships, be they intimate or those of plain friendship, profession or business. We talked about contemplation of death either personal or about that of a friend or of a member of the group. We talked about how to deal with pain, with husbands, with children. The interchanges were candid and only once in a great while were the husbands allowed to attend such a session. Bonds were created between those attending the group discussions and when one of them succumbed to her illness, all were affected but in the process they came to face their own mortality and they dealt with it with the help and support of all of them.

Sometime along the course of this program a couple of the participants opted to stop attending the regular discussions. I still followed them and treated them in my office. Some did not give me any reason for their change of mind other that they felt they no longer needed the support of the group while others explained their reasons such as the one who, much later, reminded me of that group and told me why she had left it. "I had enough trouble dealing with my own problems after mastectomy," she explained. "Without having to hear all those of the other women, neither did I feel comfortable sharing my problems with them. I became increasingly stressed as time went on until I realized what that was doing to me. I was a wreck until I decided to stop. That thing was not for me. I know most of the other women felt better after each session but it just did not work for me. And now you know."

Since I had that conversation, I always discuss the pros and cons of support groups before recommending participation. I also frequently suggest starting with a trial period of attendance for those who sound as if they might derive some benefit from it. Sharing breast cancer-associated problems may help some and may be most, but not all.

SECTION II
WEATHERING THE STORM

****

For the woman who has already gone through the primary treatment of breast cancer with its surgery followed or not by chemotherapy and radiation therapy, the news that the cancer has not been conquered, that it still inhabits her body, is the most frightening, frustrating and discouraging one. It is a source of fear and anger. Her perception is that all the effort and discomfort have been for naught. The battle is to start all over again but this time the cancer is in the advantageous position. The news is also terribly frustrating to the treating physician. It is perceived as questioning his or her skill, a setback that has to be shared with the patient. I have never been able to give such news without feeling the knot in the pit of my stomach, the sweat on the palms of my hands and the utter sense of wanting this not to be true. I can still feel my irritation at the time when, many years ago, one of my patients, no less a person than a schoolteacher, an educator, told me... to my face, that it was a well known fact that "the medical establishment" did not really want to find the cure for cancer because then "all the physicians would go out of business." I had a hard time controlling my dismay while trying to explain to this ignorant educator the researcher's glorious feeling at finding a treatment effective enough to stop albeit temporarily, the progression of a cancer in a single person let alone finding a cure for it. I had to tell my hurtful surprise at her statement and explain to her that the search for the cure was the search for human accomplishment and professional satisfaction and not for money, that the one who found it would want the entire world to know it, use it and not hide it. I had to tell her the obvious, that physicians themselves as well as members of their own families do develop cancer and do die of it as often as anyone else. Over twenty years later, one of my sons with whom I shared our oncology practice joined me for a quick lunch in my consultation room and related to me that he had, at one time, heard the exact same statement from one of his patients. Some tales and beliefs do not change.

And then how can I explain the stress of having to tell the person who was already feeling she was cured after a few months or even many years of apparent good health following the first discovery of her cancer, that it was just laying low and that it has come out of its dormancy, like the first wave of a gathering storm appearing on a peaceful-looking, lake and now requiring additional treatment. The entire process has to be explained again including the mechanism by which this can and has occur and the unpredictability and unfairness of it all.

But even more important is the explanation of the fact that this stage of the illness, bad as it may seem, is not only *treatable* but sometimes, although still rarely, it may even possibly be *curable*. If I were not an optimist and had not witnessed what can be accomplished with careful and persistent treatment of breast cancer, it would be hard to convey such optimism to the patients, their families and many times even to their family physician. I have viewed my most important role at this time as not simply to convey the bad news to the person under my care but to convey to her the true conviction that I feel that this can be helped, that the process can be stopped, slowed or even reversed for a while, whatever the length of that "while" happens to be, at the end of which other measures remain or become available to continue controlling the progression of the disease, the role to convey hope, not in a vacuum but based on facts.

Cancer recurrence can indeed be treated successfully for periods that may not be stated in advance but that, in my experience, can go sometimes longer than twenty years.

The major question that arises when breast cancer relapses is how this could happen after all that was done to try to try to eradicate it once and for all? How could it? It could because it is increasingly evident that breast cancer, while recognizable as such, is not a single disease that responds in a given way to a given form of treatment. It is a group of malignant processes all of which arise from breast tissue but that do not always look exactly the same, and even when they do they do not behave the same way and do not have the same relationship with their host, the person who harbors this cancer. It is becoming increasingly possible to identify some of these different forms of breast cancer and to apply more specific therapies.

To make that picture even more complex we have to visualize breast cancer as composed of a mixture of several of these cell lines and we have to realize that this mixture varies. If the majority of the cells making up a particular cancer happen to be sensitive to treatment "A," the bulk of that cancer will regress with that treatment even while some small components of its cell population continue to grow. Conversely if only a minority of it is sensitive to treatment "A" and is destroyed the bulk of the cancer will continue to progress since the disease as a whole follows the course of its dominant cell populations. Furthermore, it must also be understood that these cancer cells can mutate periodically thus altering their initial behavior pattern and that the proportions of these various cell populations may be altered by previous treatment. The relationship between the cancer and its host can also change and by itself cause a change in the pattern of growth. It is therefore not surprising that some of the cancers that may have already scattered some of their cells by the time they are discovered (1) may not be annihilated by the initial form of treatment and may grow in spite of it. The reason for initiating treatment early in the course of this cancer and for frequently using combinations of multiple medications is precisely for the purpose of attacking it before multiple mutations have time to occur, to attack multiple cell lines simultaneously and hopefully to allow the body's own natural defenses also to attack a smaller remaining burden of these enemy cells.

That the combination of early diagnosis and early and more effective treatment has finally met with some measure of success is evidenced by the fact that breast cancer patients' survival has increased, that the death rate from this malignancy has decreased over the years and that further decreases are anticipated.

I can picture in my mind's eyes the quizzical look I would get from the floor nurses at the hospital after I had completed the admission examination, written my notes and the treatment orders for one or the other of the very sick patients I had admitted, when I would answer their question about what I intended to do for this particular patient:

"I plan to make her well and send her home" would be my invariable answer. "I may or may not succeed but that is my plan." And these brave, patient and compassionate nurses would add an extra measure of care to those women I cared for and cared about.

The following personal conversations relate to the questions many women and men ask at the time it is discovered that the cancer has relapsed, their search for the reason of it all, their fear of the unknown, their anger at the fact that this has happened in the first place, their wish to assign some guilt for its occurrence and their quest for reassurance and help.

Read chapter: (1) DANDELION

WHAT IF IT WERE YOUR WIFE?

After giving a woman the results of the examination and tests that indicate a progression or a spread of her breast cancer and explaining the long-term implications of this illness, I always follow with a detailed presentation of the fact that this is a treatable problem. It can be stopped. It can be made to regress greatly, and many times to the point that it may *appear* to but *usually not* have completely resolved. Following this, I describe various treatment options, their relative merits and drawbacks and eventually I make a recommendation for one of them to be started.

On a number of occasions, a question comes up, usually from the husband of the patient:

"What if it were your wife, Doctor? Would you recommend that same treatment?"

And my answer has invariably been the following: "Right now I can tell you that I would recommend exactly the same as I have just recommended for your wife. However, you must understand that I am not in that situation right now. That is what I can tell you right now. If it were truly my wife I would be in a totally different situation and therefore I cannot honestly tell you whether I would be totally objective and whether I would arrive at the same recommendation. I think I would be too involved personally. While I *think* I would make the same recommendation, I would also consult a trusted colleague on that matter and have his or her evaluation, opinion and recommendation to consider very seriously. And so I both can and cannot answer your question. What I can tell you is that I have considered the course of *your* wife's illness, *her* general condition, the characteristics and previous behavior of *her* cancer as well as *her* reaction to the explanation of the treatment options I have presented. I have considered the latest information on the available forms of effective therapy and I have then made a recommendation for one of the options based upon this entire perspective. That is my best answer and that is the best I can do."

In time my wife did unfortunately develop breast cancer and I did, in fact, answer that question. We did consult colleagues I trusted and whose judgment I valued. But I also got closely involved in the management of her cancer and I did make the same recommendations as those I had made for patients unrelated to me who presented with the same clinical setting. I have been privileged and grateful for the knowledge and experience I had acquired in the field of breast cancer and therefore for the possibility of applying them to her care. Later, in my office when she talked to the women under my care she told them that she also had had surgery and radiation therapy for breast cancer and that she had been receiving adjuvant treatment. As result, they seemed to view my therapeutic recommendations with the feeling that I had a better understanding of their health problem, and I truly did.

DANDELION

The journey along the course of breast cancer is an arduous one. An understanding of the terrain ahead is very helpful while preparing to proceed along that road. Obstacles appear, adjustments have to be made around detours, accidents happen and must be dealt with. Such was the case for Joan.

Joan was 58 when this conversation occurred. She had undergone lumpectomy and radiation therapy for breast cancer three and a half years previously and now, as she was starting to feel that she was almost home free when a persistent pain developed in her lower back. She first blamed it on her recent heavy shopping expedition before the Thanksgiving holiday. Then she blamed it on the preparation of the big meal for all her guests and all the cleaning afterwards but she eventually confessed that her daughters had done most of the work and of the cleaning because she had been too achy. She just refused to acknowledge the fact that she was becoming increasingly uncomfortable with this constant pain. It is only after a month of worsening discomfort that she finally called and came to see me earlier than at her scheduled regular follow up visit.

"I know it is nothing," she started to tell me as I entered the examining room, "but you told me to call you if anything unusual happened and so here I am. I know I am crying wolf." She was trying desperately to have me confirm her wish that everything was fine.

"Everything looks and sounds fine except for the pain," I told her when I finished examining her. "Pain is pain and may be due to many causes but since you present a special situation because of your history of having had breast cancer in the past it would be wise to check further why you are having this persistent problem now."

She tried not to appear worried. "Is this truly necessary since you tell me that all is well?"

"All is not well since you have pain even though I find nothing on examination. I think you should have a bone scan and some X-ray films of your bones to start with, as well as a set of blood tests. I will see you here again four to five days after all is done."

I received the films and reports of her bone scan and corresponding X-ray films of some of her bones the day after they were done. Here they were on the viewing box in my consultation room. I could immediately see on the scan the scattering of telltale deep black dots and smudges overlying several vertebrae and ribs, confirming my suspicion and her fears. Some, although not all of the lesions seen on the scan, showed their destructive process on the X-ray films. The cancer had invaded her bones.

She was understandably upset but not completely surprised when I explained these finding to her at her visit a few days later.

"I started with breast cancer and now I have bone cancer. Isn't that a very bad one to have?" she asked.

"Bone cancer is indeed a bad one to have but you do not have bone cancer. You have breast cancer planted in your bones and that is totally different," I explained.

She appeared surprised.

"I don't understand. Isn't bone cancer the same as cancer in the bone? How can I have breast cancer in the bone?"

"I explained that to you a long time ago when your first came to consult me after your surgery but I will explain it to you again in a simple way: Assume that your body is a property with a house and a lawn. On the lawn grows nice uniform Kentucky blue grass. One day as you look at it you notice a patch of dandelion in a corner of the lawn. That is the equivalent of a cancer for that lawn. You quickly look around and see no other dandelions. Assuming it is the only patch on the lawn you dig it out roots and all. This is the same as when the cancerous lump was removed from your breast. You actually dig out some extra ground around it for good measure in order to make sure that no little root extensions or small seeds have been left behind. This is the same as the wide excision and node removal from the armpit that were performed after the initial excision of the breast lump."

"For even better measure of control you burn the ground immediately around that area with one of these weed blow torches because you know that little dandelion seeds may frequently be present in the vicinity of the more obvious growth and rather than make a bigger ugly hole there you just burn it. This is the same as the radiation therapy after the lumpectomy rather than a mastectomy."

"Then what? Then if you have noticed the presence of tiny little dandelions around the main one when you examine closely the big clump of soil you removed around it or if the dandelion's flower had already become fuzzy with its flying seeds you worry about the possibility that some of the seeds might have been carried away by wind or rain to other parts of your lawn, garden or property. These seeds are too small to be seen. Furthermore, even if they have scattered most of them do not survive. They either dry out, get eaten by the birds, the ants or the worms, fall where the soil is not suitable for their survival or growth and they disintegrate. A few however may survive where they have fallen and there, in time, they mature and sprout new *dandelions*. Whether these grow in the rose patch or in the geranium box on the third floor window it is still *dandelion*, not hay or chickweed. This is the same process as the spread of cancer. The initial lump and surrounding tissues have been removed but if some of the cells had already separated and traveled through the blood stream some of these cells may have survived the attack of your immune system and eventually grew anywhere they have settled, just as the dandelion seeds did. You may even have spread a weed killer for good measure on your lawn, the equivalent of a course of chemotherapy after the initial treatment of the breast cancer but even that may not have prevented altogether the later growth of some of the surviving resistant seeds or cells. If and when these cells grow they grow as *breast* cancer deposits or metastases regardless of whether this growth takes place in bone or any other tissue. Treatment is therefore directed against breast cancer, not bone cancer in that case. On the lawn a type of weed killer specifically capable of killing dandelion is used, not one used specifically against the lawn grass, and it is sprayed all over the property. Similarly in the case of breast cancer found to have spread in bone or any other tissue, medications capable of killing breast cancer tissue are used. The treatment is not directed specifically to bone or to lung or liver, it is directed against breast cancer cell deposits wherever they may be located in the body. The medications are administered internally, orally or by injection, and circulate all over the body in all its tissues."

"Now I understand," she said. "I also understand that when I was told that my aunt who had breast cancer died later of liver cancer it was not a different cancer as I thought, it was still breast cancer which had spread in her liver. What I have is still bad though, isn't it?"

"Yes, it is bad but not half as bad as bone cancer arising from bone. Breast cancer spread into bone can be very treatable and can respond very well to specific treatment. I have great hopes to get this back under control and you should feel very positive about it."

I tried to be and to sound reassuring but how reassuring can one be while explaining to a person that her cancer is still active, even though treatable, after a three and a half year period of quiescence?

"Can you make it go away?" she then asked.

"Like in make-it-go-away-never-to-come-back, no. It can improve, it can regress and your pain may improve greatly or even may go away completely. Only time will tell if the treatment will work that way but, as I already told you, there is a very good chance that it will."

"What if the treatment does not work or if after a while the cancer becomes resistant to the treatment? Will that be it for me...curtains?" She made a gesture as if cutting her neck with her extended fingers while sticking out the tip of her tongue and popping her eyes at the same time. She was always a bit of a comedian and even under unhappy circumstances such as on that day that trait always came out.

I shook my head. "Not at all. Fortunately, there are many forms of treatment that may control the growth of the cancer or make it regress. In your case, hormonal treatment will be the best choice. If it does not work for you or when it stops working other forms of treatment will be applied. You must understand that the treatment of breast cancer, or of any cancer for that matter, has not been cast in stone ten years ago. There are already many well-established and effective forms of treatment, new ways of applying old treatments, new treatments, new combinations and constantly ongoing research into new methods of therapy. That is the reason why we oncologists treat breast cancer even when we know that the treatment benefits are of finite duration, a duration that may not be predicted at the outset. Tomorrow, next week, next month or in six months something new and different will become available and may give us all additional time and additional comfort. Because of this I don't give up easily and neither should you. I plan that this will work out and I will do my best to make it so, I promise you."

"At least I have some hope. I would like to go on for a while. I have a lot to live for and I want to live."

Hope. It is not an empty word. Hope is the most important item the oncologist carries and shares with patients and their families. Hope is not only what keeps the patient going it is just as importantly what also maintains the physician's determination to go on treating and trying to maintain life and comfort.

If I had not acknowledged and believed deeply in that hope, I would never had lasted in my profession. Hope for the oncologist is like a chess game. Even when he scores by taking a knight or a horseman, he knows the next move is his crafty opponent's. He has to start thinking, "how can I maintain this advantage and, if I lose it, what will my next move be, what will be the move after that one and the ones after and after that?" All along strategy is planned and strategy is constantly modified because the enemy's moves cannot always be predicted. But the hope to win, to end in a draw or to stall the final checkmate as long as possible persists throughout the contest. Hope.

My younger son who is now an oncologist has summarized his work with metastatic cancer in the following statement: "My patient has to pay what is equivalent to a very large income tax, the ultimate end of progressive cancer. I, the oncologist am like the accountant and, while I cannot eliminate that tax, I can keep filing for extensions with one treatment or another as long as possible while at the same time keeping abreast of the changes in the available treatments, the equivalents to the changing tax laws of cancer."

MORE HORMONAL
TREATMENT? FOR ME?

George sounded incredulous. "First, I could not believe I had breast cancer, and then I could not understand how this could affect my bones although now I do after you explained it all to me (1). Now you tell me I need more hormonal treatment. Is there any of it still available after the one I have been taking."

George was in his early seventies when this conversation took place. By the time his breast cancer had finally been diagnosed it had been there for a while and was growing. After the surgery he had undergone more than three years previously I had given him hormonal adjuvant treatment because the cancer, although still localized, had reached a stage at which there was a serious likelihood that it might have already spread its microscopic implants elsewhere in the body and, in the hope that if it were so, the treatment might delay or even prevent the growth of these suspected metastases. Tests performed on the tumor had shown it to be potentially sensitive to hormonal treatment. He had also already received a combination of non-hormonal anticancer medications. He had been well for almost four years.

"Do you remember when I explained to you that your breast cancer was fairly extensive when it was first found three years ago and that it has been tested and found to be what is termed hormone receptor positive?"

"Yes. That is why you prescribed the hormonal treatment, for prevention."

"Well, but I explained to you that this was not prevention as most people chose to call it. It is in fact treatment of suspected but undetectable microscopic seeding of the cancer cells in parts of the body away from the breast where they had originated."

71

"Yes, I remember. I guess it did not work."

"May be and may be not. It is certain now that what was suspected when your first came to me was indeed there. The microscopic spread of the cancer had already taken place. It is possible that it has grown in spite of the hormonal treatment and the other chemotherapy. It is also possible that the treatment is the reason why is has taken it that long to appear in the bones where it had already planted itself and that without this it might have appeared much earlier. Still, the fact remains that this cancer was strongly hormone receptor positive, meaning sensitive to certain hormonal changes that can be induced in the body. Because of this the treatment of choice is still that of hormonal treatment. It is not the only form of treatment but it is the most effective in this setting in addition to being the one associated with a better quality of life."

"So what do you recommend?"

George was pragmatic. He did not waste time with words. I guess that it why he had been successful businessman. He would get the information, evaluate the problem, ask a few very pertinent questions and then decide what should be done and when. That is how he approached his own health problem: "What do we do now?"

"I have to start by telling you that breast cancer behaves very much the same way in men as it does in women. In young women, as you may have heard, when it is spread in the body through metastases, a hormone sensitive breast cancer will frequently improve if the production of estrogens, the female hormones, is suppressed."

"Yes, I know that. I remember hearing that sometimes the ovaries are removed to stop the growth of the cancer."

"That is indeed sometimes the fastest and most effective way to control this type of breast cancer. There are also other ways of suppressing the production of hormones by the ovaries by means of medications. Many years ago at the Memorial Sloan-Kettering Cancer Center it was discovered that the same basic type of treatment worked in men. There, however, it was the removal of the source of male hormones which produced the best regressions of breast cancer metastases." I waited for the expected reaction.

"Oh." He suddenly appeared worried.

"Yeah!" I shook my head affirmatively. "It was found at the time that the surgical removal of the testes was the fastest method of stopping the production of male hormones and the most effective way of frequently causing the regression of breast cancer metastases in males."

"Removing my testicles?" Now he was really worried.

"Yes. But of course it is not the only way although it is the most rapidly effective. If it works the relief of all the bone pains you have been complaining of for the past several weeks will occur quite rapidly. It is sometimes immediate although most of the time it does take a few weeks and it occurs gradually."

"Boy! This is a bit of a shock, you know."

He was truly rattled but there was no other way of putting it.

"Yes I know, but let me ask you something. Are you sexually active at all at this time?"

"No, not for at least the past three years, not since the chemotherapy. Even for some time before that my sexual activity had been... how should I put it... sporadic at best. We are not youngsters you know. My wife is sixty-eight and I am seventy-one and in pain. Come to think of it losing my testicles would not make much of a difference on that score. Still, I need a little time to think about this." He smiled and added: "I am still sentimentally attached to my equipment although it has been on the shelf for quite a while."

"Of course. But, as I started to say earlier, surgery is not the only option. There are medications administered by mouth and/or by injection that can accomplish the same result. It means of course taking tablets daily and /or receiving injections monthly. These same medications are used in the treatment of prostate cancer. Side effects may occur but are usually quite tolerable. The effect on sexual function is the same as with the surgery but as we discussed it, in your situation this is not a real problem anyway. Interestingly enough, since cost is the universal buzzword in medicine nowadays, the cost of the medicinal treatment is probably higher in the long run that the cost of the surgery. Either one of the two methods would be a good first choice."

That had been difficult to deal with. I am still struck about the ease with which physicians over the years have been able to recommend the surgical removal of the ovaries to young women with advanced breast cancer and how difficult it has been for them to recommend the equivalent surgical castration to men with metastatic cancer of the prostate or of the breast. Male physician dominance and empathy with the male patients are the obvious unconscious mechanism of this emotional dichotomy.

"What about chemotherapy?" he asked. "Is it not an option?"

"Chemotherapy would not be my first choice at the present time because it is associated with more toxic side effects and because hormonal therapy is more likely to be effective. There are also other forms of hormonal treatment available. The one I explained is the more effective for your present condition and there are others. It may be necessary to give you some radiation therapy to painful areas of your bones along the way but it does not appear urgent now since your pain medications seem to have been quite helpful. Let me know at any time if the pain gets worse or is not helped by your pain pills. I can always do something to help relieve it. There is no need for you to suffer. The best relief will of course occur if the cancer regresses with treatment. There is also sometimes a temporary increase in pain at the onset of treatment but it is temporary.

George decided to talk all this over with his wife and think about it for few days. I told him to have her call me if she had any questions.

"Needless to say," he added, "I am not happy at all about this and by this I mean that the cancer is still with me. But thanks again for explaining it all to me. It is easier for me to arrive at a decision if I know the facts. Now tell me what will happen once I have the surgery or take the hormonal medications. I understand it is not a cure but what happens after that?"

"George," I said, "indeed this is not a cure. If this treatment is effective you may look forward to experiencing good and even complete relief of your pain, possibly for a long period of time along with healing of the lesions in your bones or anywhere they may be present. If it works...fine. If or when it becomes obvious that it has not been effective or is no longer effective then a different course will have to be started. Even if it does cause the cancer to regress causing your condition to improve you, unfortunately, cannot expect this improvement to go on forever. It is finite in that it may last a few weeks, months or even several years sometimes but the improvement will eventually come to an end and a different treatment will have to be considered at that time."

"Then it is also possible that if I opt for surgery I may have undergone the procedure for nothing".

"That is indeed and unfortunately true and certainly something to think about."

"Hmm! Food for thought" he added. He thought for a while, then "How will you know that it is improving or that it is worsening at any time," he asked.

"I will have to monitor you fairly closely in the beginning and at longer intervals once it is established that you are doing well. You will still have to be checked regularly."

"Well now, I have a lot of thinking and of planning to do. At least I know what I am up against, not that I did not suspect it, and I also see a hopeful plan of action as limited as it may be. Still, the idea of that surgery knocked me out for a loop!"

"We will take it one step at a time George and I plan that it will go well and so should you. I have already told you that medicinal treatment for hormonal suppression is still a good and effective alternative."

He called the next day with more of the same questions and to announce his decision to go ahead with the surgery. He did very well after the surgery. His pain improved very rapidly. The regression of the cancer was confirmed by the X-ray follow up.

The improvement lasted almost two years during which he continued to work part time, he traveled with his wife, visited his two children and his grandchildren in Oregon and California several times. He tried to take advantage of that period of respite from his cancer. He led an active social life whenever he could.

When the next relapse occurred, another good response to treatment occurred but was much shorter. Eventually, he refused further chemotherapy after he had received several additional courses the last of which had made him quite uncomfortable without producing any worthwhile relief. Both he and his wife expressed their feeling of gratitude for the quality time they had been able to spend together and during which they were able to experience the joys of grand-parenthood while leaving many memories of George with their grandchildren. Radioisotope therapy, external radiation and pain medications relieved his discomfort during his final few months and he finally died peacefully at home as he had wished it.

DON'T TELL HER

Should one tell the bad news and all the bad news when cancer progresses and health deteriorates as a consequence? Is there room for some white lies, some unrealistic measure of optimism, some glossing over the bad news and balancing it with a light of hope everlasting? The physicians who treat cancer patients are often confronted with these questions.

When, on the day of her first consultation at my office, Beatrice Goldstein left my consultation room to go to the examining room, her brother stayed a moment longer with me. As soon as she was out of sight and of earshot he got close to me and, glancing sideways toward where she has entered the examining room, he whispered, "Whatever you tell her, don't mention to her that the cancer has spread. It would be terrible."

"In what way? Has she mentioned anything to you about this probability?" I asked.

"No, but I know how she would take it. Believe me. I know her. She is my sister," he protested.

"Well then, what do you think I should tell her?" I could easily predict his answer.

"Tell her she has some type of inflammation in her bones or her joints, that you will give her a treatment for it... anything... but please..."

"Your sister, I see, is a retired high school principal. She is highly educated. She probably reads at least one newspaper daily and watches current events reports on TV. Do you really think I can pull the wool over her eyes?" He looked increasingly worried. "Personally," I continued, "I don't think I can, and I don't think I should try," I added. "I can easily lie to her and hope that I can remember these lies at each of the following visits. I may then have to tell more lies and even that may well be manageable."

He did not know what I was driving at and still looked worried.

"Well that is fine then. At least she will not have to worry."

"Not that simple," I went on. "Even if she truly believes whatever stories I can concoct, somewhere along the way, one good day the entire pack of lies will hit us all in the face and will hit her the hardest. Someone will slip, at a lab, when taking an X-ray, during conversation or by leaving a record or a report on a table or such similar thing. The impact will be devastating to her and will certainly wreck her relationship with her treating physician, be it me or anyone else. No. Lying is not a solution. I prefer to be the one to tell her the truth because I can tell it in a constructive way, a way acceptable to her, all the while emphasizing the hopeful aspects of the treatment."

He was getting exasperated. "I don't see how you can do this," he went on.

"Don't misunderstand me. I don't plan to hit her with it between the eyes so to speak. I don't do that. But I will not lie to her. I will find out what she knows and will see how much she is prepared to hear. Has she been told anything by her surgeon?" I asked.

"Not really," he told me. "He explained that he had requested to be informed of the results of her tests as soon as they were completed. When he received the report of the bone scan that was done because of her pains, he told her she had some arthritis as well as other problems with her bones and he advised her to come and see you. He told *me* that the breast cancer has spread into her bones and that the outlook was bad."

"And what did you tell her?" I asked.

"I could not tell her that! I told her everything would be all right, that it was not serious but that we should go for the consultation anyway. What else could I tell her?"

"That's all right for now," I told him. "I just wanted to know what she had been told in order to be able to take it from there. Why don't you sit in the waiting room until I finish examining her and then I will call you back in as soon as that is done We will all talk together."

During the examination I spotted a few tender areas over the spine and ribs but Mrs. Goldstein, other than responding whenever I found a tender spot, made neither comments nor asked any questions.

"I want to tell you a couple of things before you talk to both of us together," she finally said when I had completed the examination. "I have to know what is happening to me. Please understand that I can deal with the truth and cannot stand being left in the dark. I know that my brother is very concerned and tries to protect me but this is my problem and I am the one who has to deal with it." It was immediately obvious to me that this intelligent and perceptive lady already knew what had happened to her and was setting up the rules of our relationship.

"OK, I understand and that is the way I always prefer to handle this. Join us in my office once you are dressed. Take your time."

When she came into my consultation room a few minutes later her brother joined us and we all settled in our chairs for the "conversation."

"What did Dr. Shapiro tell you when he referred you to me?" I asked.

"He said I had some arthritis in my back and possibly some other problem with my bones and that I should come to see you."

"Well, what problems do you think you have other than the arthritis?"

"I have had arthritis and pain in my back on and off for a long time, Doctor. This feels different. I think my cancer has spread in my bones. That is what I think," she said looking at her brother.

"You are right," I said as I glanced at him and went back to address her. "I have looked at your bone scan, at the X-ray films and all the other tests you have had recently. There is indeed quite a bit of arthritis, in your back particularly, but in addition there is also definite evidence that the cancer has spread to several spots in the bones. On my examination there is no evidence of any other spread at present and that is good."

Mr. Fine, her brother, had been sitting stiffly upright in this armchair looking at his sister for some terrible reaction but observing none he finally relaxed and leaned back. No charades were being played any longer. We were now exchanging information and advice.

"How bad is this?" she asked.

"It is bad," I explained, "because it shows that the cancer had already spread at the time of the initial surgery but was not apparent because the spread was microscopic. Still, it was thought that you were at a relatively elevated risk of such problem occurring in the future and that is why you were started on adjuvant hormonal treatment. Compared to some other types of breast cancer behavior this is a better one to have because it appears limited to bones and has progressed quite slowly. Indeed, it has taken it 4 years since your initial surgery to manifest itself. It is also likely that the hormonal treatment has been instrumental in delaying it recurrence. Based on that I can tell you that it is very likely to improve with other hormonal treatment. As things stand today it is not going to be cured, but it is very likely to improve so let's get going with the treatment that, at this time, is very simple: here is a prescription for another hormonal medication which acts somewhat differently from the one you already had. It has a good track record of effectiveness against breast cancer in a setting such as yours. Start taking it daily. In addition, I will also start a treatment with a medication given intravenously over a two hours period monthly. That one works by making bone tissue less vulnerable to the damage caused by breast cancer. It is neither an anticancer chemotherapy nor a hormonal medication. It works specifically on bone tissue and not on the cancer and generally has no side effects. My secretary will give you a series of appointments for this as well as for a re-examination in four to six weeks but call at anytime in between if you have any questions or problems."

We went on to discuss potential side effects, treatment alternatives and the possibility of radiation therapy.

"Thank you, Doctor," she said at the end. "Thank you for being straight forward with me. I am not happy about my situation but I understand that I may do well with the treatment. I want to do well. I have a lot to live for, many things I still want to do and so I hope you will keep me going for a long time."

"I fully intend to," I said. "I will do the best I know and the best I can to keep you well."

As they walked out of the consultation room, her brother grabbed both of my hands. "I don't know how you do it or how you can do that day after day, but I thank you," he said.

I was always able to "do it" but not always able to do it with impunity. For years I kept antacid tablets in my desk drawers for daytime use and on my night table to be chewed as needed through the night. It took me years to make peace with the fact that I should not and could not take over and constantly feel the emotional reactions of those who came to consult me with their cancer and who waited to hear from me the words that, in their minds, would seal the fate of their body and of their life. I had to find ways to tell the truth, often enough the happy truth, frequently the terrible truth, many times most of, if not the whole truth, but enough of it to be informative, in an acceptable, non-traumatic way while at the same time conveying hope, all of it without rehearsal, and under new sets of circumstances each time. The words had to be right the first time. Once out, like the genie of the bottle, they could not be erased, neither could their impact be softened. I could not lie because lies have to be remembered lest they fly back at you and hit you in the face at the most unexpected and most inopportune moment. I tried to spare as much as possible those who came asking for hope and bore holes in my stomach at night and woke me up in the morning with sore joints.

This process reminds me often of a word game we played as kids. The name of the game was "the prosecutor." One of the players was chosen to be the "prosecutor" and could ask any question of any of the other players who were the "accused." Answers were to be always truthful but certain words could not be used, words like "yes," "no," "black," "white," "Mr.," "Mrs.," and "Miss." The "prosecutor" would try to trip the "accused" he questioned into using one of these words in their answers. Three mistakes and the "accused" was put away out of the game. The skill was both in the ability to frame the questions and the finesse in answering truthfully through the careful choice of paraphrases without uttering the forbidden words. On many occasions in my work, I found myself in the position of the "accused" of that game, having to tell the truth without using the forbidden words and yet without ever lying.

In time I learned to contemplate my own attitudes. I slowly developed the ability to give all the support, the care the consolations, the explanations, with all the time and patience it took, but without taking on the suffering at the same time. I seldom got upset at being awakened by calls at night, or at being asked questions which may have appeared inept but which had been very troubling to the patient or to the family member who called. I still may get upset and lose patience very briefly at times, but then after all we are all human although the physician is still frequently perceived and expected to be above these weaknesses of everyday life.

I relaxed my whole being, stopped having heartburn at night (although it still occurs sometimes during the day) or sore joints in the morning after tossing and turning all night. I have come to the realization that very few situations in life are worth becoming sick over. Problems are to be resolved and not to become anxious about. I also found during my sleepless nights of quiet introspection that solutions may be sought in several directions, that some are not acceptable and require a substitute, that the most effective is not always the best for a given situation, that given the same illness, at the same stage, different persons must be treated differently, that compromises have to be made and to be accepted, that a questioning patient is not to be seen as challenging one but as one requesting needed information in order to help her or him to arrive at her or his own decisions and compromises.

For many years now, I have shunned serious plays and movies and have emphasized comedy. I exchange jokes and funny stories with my patients. Life spent side by side with cancer is hard enough for both patient and physician. It is harder for the one with cancer and it is tension producing for the treating physician. Truth made acceptable through its explanation, decreases both fear and tension. A little humor relaxes everyone. Laughter is indeed good and effective medicine.

I TELL EVERYONE

Truth about a given patient's condition can often best emanate from the patient herself in response to questions expressed or implied by family, friends or others who interact with her.

Evelyn was a good example of such a situation. She had just joined the breast cancer discussion group I had started for a group of women receiving chemotherapy under my care. She was sixty-four and had metastatic breast cancer for which she had just started a new course of chemotherapy. She turned out to be the most positive person in the entire group.

We would meet once a week at 6:00 PM in a small conference room of the hospital and the eight or ten women would vent their problems with life under the pall of breast cancer and its treatment. Many times, they offered information that they had not given me in the course of their treatment and follow up at my office. The informal format of these meetings around coffee and cake facilitated the interaction.

"I tell everyone, all my friends, about my cancer and found out this way that I helped them as much as I helped myself," Evelyn started telling us one evening.

Everyone around her stopped talking and listened as she sat very straight on her chair because of her backache. She had a twinkle in her brown eyes and a smiling face framed by the short "salt and pepper" hair of her well-fitted wig.

"Yes," she added, "I found that when it became obvious that my cancer was advancing my friends became increasingly reluctant to come and visit me as before. These were my good and close friends and I soon noticed that our telephone conversations had become generally

82

shorter. They avoided talking about my health. Their dwelled mostly on unimportant matters and even sounded uneasy talking to me. I realized that while they were still good friends they did not know how to address my problem and so they avoided it and avoided me at the same time. But I found a solution to this situation. I started calling two or three of them at a time and would invite them to come to my house and have coffee and cake with me the way we had done it for years until we almost stopped doing it in recent months. They could not refuse, and when they came I immediately opened and closed the subject by telling them that the treatment of my cancer was progressing well, that I was coming along. Then, very slowly and timidly, they started asking questions and talking about it and I found all of them to be truly concerned and supportive once they found out that I was not upset by that topic. We would then go on with our coffee, tea, cake and talk as we always had. They realized they were not hurting me because I was so happy to see them all as always. They very quickly began to feel at ease and we were again able to talk freely about everything as before including the new topic of my cancer. We are back visiting by telephone or by meeting together without the fear of a conversational 'faux pas.' Now when they come I say: 'my cancer is doing fine, let us play canasta'. We all laugh and go on with the visit."

She had told this entire story almost in one breath. All were silent for a while. Many had shaken their heads affirmatively from time to time during her statement as if to signify that they had also experienced some of the same reactions among their friends.

This brave lady had discovered very early a disturbance in her social relationships the cause of which she recognized intuitively. She then undertook to correct it immediately and energetically. The thing she had discovered was that she was the one who had to help her friends, even her close friends, to come to grips with her illness. She gave them her help and they gave her theirs and that friendship sustained all of them.

Since that time people's perception of cancer have changed and cancer has, so to speak, come out of the closet. It is more readily acknowledged and openly discussed more so in our country than in Europe where physicians still tend to be more paternalistic with their patients in their conversations about it.

TRUST

As the journey along the way of breast cancer proceeds, obstacles appear, frightening obstacles. Can the leader be trusted to steer safely trough? Should a new and more reliable one be sought?

"Not that we don't trust you..." he started to say.

As soon as I heard the beginning of the sentence I knew what would follow. I had finished informing the patient and her husband of the recently discovered fact that her cancer had reached a new phase and that I was about to recommend a new treatment plan. Trust in my skills was obviously going to be questioned.

Celia had undergone a right mastectomy for a rather large breast cancer associated with metastases in many of the lymph nodes of the armpit. She had received adjuvant chemotherapy for a whole year at the time and had remained well for eight in spite of the poor prognosis that was based on the initial findings. Eventually, she would come to see me about once or twice a year for follow up.

At the time of her most recent visit a small mass had been detected at the base of her neck. The biopsy had confirmed the presence of a metastatic deposit in that location and subsequently chest films had revealed the presence of multiple nodules in both lungs. She had no symptoms but her husband had already called for the results of the tests. I had informed him of the findings and of the need for systemic treatment with anticancer medications. That day's visit at my office was for the purpose of reviewing her clinical course that had been rather benign over several years and to outline and explain the proposed course of treatment.

I explained the pathology report, both the original one of the mastectomy and that of the recent biopsy including the hormone receptor data for each. I discussed the X-ray findings and the blood tests. Finally I explained the fact that the appearance of metastases after that long a delay since the original diagnosis meant that the cancer was fortunately not a terribly aggressive one and that it had a very good chance of responding well to the proposed treatment. I then waited for the next question. I had found out over the years of treating cancer patients that there is some essential information that must be given at the outset. Other information is frequently best withheld until the patient has assimilated the first and is ready to tackle more. That is when the next question and the ones that follow are formulated. At such times, answers, I found, are best formulated explicitly but also best limited to respond to the specifically requested information.

There was a moment of silence. "Does that mean that the cancer will go away?" Mr. G. finally asked. I then proceeded to explain the implications of the appearance of the metastases. "At that stage of the disease, while one could hope for regression of the malignant process, the likelihood of a permanent cure was, at best, infinitesimal." I then went on to recommend a particular course of treatment as well as the reasons why I had picked that particular one. I described its potential benefits, limitations, side effects and risks.

"Only time will tell whether this treatment will work the way I hope," I told them. "In your case, it is very likely to be effective because of the time it has taken that cancer to show up its spread but still we will have to wait and see. I think it is worth a good try. Mind you," I added, "this is not the only effective treatment. There are number of alternative single or combinations of medications which can be as effective." And I went on to explain that the recommendation I had made was based on the combined evaluation of its effectiveness, tolerance in terms of toxicity, and ease of administration compared to the others.

I recommended to both Celia and her husband to think about what I had told them although not to defer their decision too long because, given the extend and the location of the disease, it was not advisable to delay the onset of treatment.

Celia had remained silent throughout the discussion, visibly upset at this turn of events after so many years but also appearing somewhat ill at ease. As I awaited some type of response or reaction for a moment after I had finished talking, Mr. G. broke the silence somewhat hesitantly.

"Not that we don't trust you doctor after so many years," he managed to say, "but my wife feels she would like to have another opinion. We talked about it with her cousin who knows an oncologist at Mt Sinai whom she wants her to consult. I hope you understand." He sounded almost apologetic.

This was not the first time I had encountered this response to the news of another crisis in the course of this illness. Something in their attitude had led me to expect it from the moment they had come into my consultation room to talk to me. I hurried to reassure them and to tell them that it was perfectly understandable.

"Two heads are better than one," I replied, "and I feel this is a good idea."

They appeared relieved.

"You have taken good care of me all along," Celia added, "but my cousin insisted that I go to see this oncologist and has already made an appointment with her for me. I hope you understand. She has been like a sister to me and is very concerned about what has happened, and after all it is my life."

"Please don't worry Mrs. G. You must feel that you have explored all the avenues of treatment you and your family want. Please tell me the name of the doctor you are going to consult and I will make sure to send her at once all the information she may need in order to evaluate your condition and to advise you on the treatment she will recommend."

The name she gave was that of a colleague I knew and respected and I told her so.

"Your cousin had made an excellent choice of consultant," I told her. "I know this doctor quite well and we have shared in the care of many patients in the past. You could not be in better hands. If after your consultation you want to return here for your treatment, please give me a call and I will prepare everything to get started. I you decide to continue under her care please let me know. In that case, I know that you will be well taken care of and I will wish you the best."

I had the feeling she would not return to my care. I felt frustrated at the thought that a person for whom I had tried and was again trying my best to control the growth of a lethal cancer had lost her confidence in my skill, experience and knowledge at the time when that confidence was essential to her care.

There is no greater satisfaction for a physician in that field of medicine than the feeling that as a result of his or her efforts a patient improves and tells him or her that she feels so much better. The sight of side by side X-ray films or scans confirming the diminution or disappearance of a cancerous lesion following treatment is the source of indescribable joy as is the sadness at the sight of progression of the illness. Being placed in a position of having to stop in mid-fight like in this situation is a letdown with an unavoidable after taste of rejection and, worse, possibly of failure. It is one of the sources of the constant self-scrutiny to which we have to subject ourselves, that which frequently keeps us awake at night, that which tempers our feeling of omnipotence and imposes upon us a necessary measure of humility.

THE MESSAGE

Rose was a grade school teacher in her early fifties. She was short and plump with a pleasant round face and hair pulled up in an old fashion but becoming, loose bun. She had been referred to me because having undergone a right mastectomy for breast cancer six years earlier she had recently started to develop aches and pains everywhere. The pain had progressed to the point where she had become unable to move around without severe discomfort. After the initial consultation I had hospitalized her for tests to be followed by appropriate treatment.

Her X-ray films, done that day, had confirmed my clinical impression of extensive spread of the cancer to the bones. I came to see her that evening after my office hours and after having reviewed the films in the Radiology department of the hospital. I arrived at her bedside during visiting hours while her husband was still there. This was the opportunity to inform both of them of the findings and of the treatment plan.

As I sat on the empty chair beside her husband she addressed me immediately, as a schoolteacher would one of her students:

"Have your checked all my results Doctor?"

"Yes," I replied dutifully. "As a matter of fact I have just reviewed all your films and all the blood test results and I have come to explain to you all the findings."

"Good! My husband is here Doctor and is listening and I want you to tell me truthfully what I have. I have to know the truth. You must tell me."

"You know you had a cancer in your breast when you had the mastectomy four years ago."

"Yes."

"Well, sometimes some cancer cells leave the initial tumor in the breast before it is found and removed and they plant themselves in other places in the body. They frequently settle in the bones but these nests are microscopic at first and undetectable. They cause absolutely no symptoms and may cause none for a long time. They may grow slowly over months and years and then eventually produce enough damage to cause symptoms. That is what has happened to you. Fortunately, this type of spread of breast cancer frequently responds to hormonal treatment and it is this type of treatment that I recommend for it. It has a very good chance of causing your bones to heal and your pain to improve."

"Are you telling me that I have cancer in my bones?" she then asked anxiously.

In keeping with her initial request and instructions, I replied that this was unfortunately true but I added that as I had already told them both this type of cancer spread was very likely to improve with treatment even though this treatment would not cure it completely but that it was not unusual for the improvement to last sometimes several years."

She appeared stunned for a while. Her husband held her hand as she cried. We talked more about the actual treatment and I left them once she had calmed down. I stopped at the nurses' station and left some medication orders for her.

The next evening at about the same time I stopped to see her and again her husband was with her.

She appeared no longer upset or anxious and I thought that she had accepted both her diagnosis and my words of reassurance and encouragement. Was I surprised then when I heard her words of greeting?

"Good evening doctor," she said, "I hope that you now have all the results of my tests and that you can tell me what I have. My husband is here with me and you must tell us both what is going on with me."

For a brief moment I was puzzled. Was I dreaming or had we already had this conversation? Then I quickly realized she was somehow, unconsciously, conveying a message to me. She really had not wanted to hear the previous day's bad news. She wanted to hear that things were not that bad and that she would get better.

I don't believe in lying to someone whose confidence I absolutely need in order to carry out the treatment as it should be. I needed her cooperation in this endeavor. Cooperation meant knowledge and understanding. I don't believe either in hitting someone over the head with such a diagnosis particularly when she was telling me quite clearly, although subliminally, that she wanted neither to recall nor to hear again the previous day's version I had given her of the truth. She had promptly buried it in the deepest recess of her memory and had hidden the key in that cache where she would have a hard time finding it herself. I had to find the non-threatening but truthful answer immediately.

"All right," I said, "let me explain it to you simply: You have had a cancer of the breast in the past and some women who have had breast cancer may develop a problem with their bones months or years later. This particular problem, when it occurs, is manifest by the appearance of scattered areas of loss of calcium from the bones. It weakens them in these areas and causes pain... and that is what you have. Fortunately this type of calcium loss can frequently be reversed by hormonal treatment and that is the treatment I recommend for you. I think you will do well with it."

I then went on to explain how this would be done, which side effects could occur and how the follow up of her condition would proceed. I added that if for some reason there would be no improvement with this medication or should it eventually fail after a good response, several other forms of treatment were available and one of them would be substituted for it. She did not ask any more details and, in this particular case, I knew better that to provide information that was not requested of me at that time.

"Do you have any other questions about this?" I finally asked.

There was a look of relief on her face. "No," she said, "thank you, thank you very much".

Did I tell her the truth? Yes.

Did I tell her the whole truth that second time? Yes and no.

Did I do the right thing? I think so.

The lesson I learnt on that occasion for my own education was: listen first and very carefully before you talk, then keep listening just as carefully while you are talking.

Still, this experience raised many questions in my mind.

Under similar circumstances is the truth what I state it to be? Should the stated truth about the course of an illness or its treatment not change or adapt to the problem? And therefore what I state to be true may not necessarily be what someone else believes it to be. Is the whole truth the only truth?

I believe that an acknowledgement of a certain degree of ignorance is also an important part of the truth and that some proffered truths are lies.

Finally, I have come to the conclusion that truth as it is requested by a person looking desperately for some hope in life with cancer, is sometimes best expressed as a mixture of well established facts in a context of an acknowledged level of ignorance with a positive but cautious measure of hope rather than as the devastating and often simplified statement of what one has condensed from a mountain of extremely varied information.

THIS IS IT

When all seems lost because of a set back, when the future looks bleak, when it looks like there is no hope anymore, take a deep breath, step back for a moment and remember the words of the famous ball player: "it's not over until..." And so it was when Elaine asked: "What did my CAT scan show?"

"You just brought in the films with you," I protested, "I have not yet had a chance to look at them. Let me first finish with your examination and I will look at them with you right in my office."

She was so anxious I decided not to wait. I opened the X-ray envelope in the examining room and pulled out the films one by one. Once the films were hanging on the viewing box I quickly identified those rows of pictures that gave the clearest images of the liver. There they were. The multiple gray spots that stood out against the homogeneous background of the liver and indicated the presence of tumor deposits scattered in that large organ.

"Well? What is the verdict?"

"You are innocent," I said, trying to lighten up the conversation. "There is no verdict. There is a diagnosis. These pictures show that your liver is a little damaged."

"Damaged by what? By the cancer? I knew it when the doctor at the radiology lab would not tell me what he saw and told me I could bring you the films to look at after he had finished reading them. This is it then! There is nothing that can be done for liver cancer. How long do I have? I am terminal? Oh my God! What will I tell my husband? What will I tell my daughter?"

"Wait," I said, "who said anything about being terminal or that there is nothing that can be done? Hold everything. Let me finish examining you and then we will sit in my office and talk. One thing I will tell you right away now. There is treatment for this and so don't go to buy a shovel and don't start digging the hole yet. There's a lot of life in you and so don't you give it up prematurely."

Elaine was in her mid-fifties and her breast cancer had been diagnosed shortly after her husband had finally recovered from a severe heart attack. Her story was one I had heard many times. She had been aware of the breast mass for a while but argued that she had been too busy taking care of her sick husband and had chosen to overlook this lump until after he was well on his way to recovery. Her cancer was already quite extensive in both the breast and the lymph nodes when she finally consulted her physician and underwent surgery. She had received chemotherapy for six months and had been maintained on hormonal therapy until now, for almost two years. And now this: liver metastases.

Her examination completed she got dressed and came into my small consultation office. She had come in alone.

"Where is your husband?" I asked.

"In the waiting room."

"I will call him in."

She hesitated a moment and then, "OK," she said.

I buzzed my secretary on the intercom and asked her to show him into my office. As soon as he came in, she told him: "The CAT scan shows that I have liver cancer."

I immediately interrupted:

"You do not have liver cancer. You have breast cancer planted in the liver and that is totally different. Let me explain all that to you. As you may remember your breast cancer was quite large when it was found and it had already invaded several lymph nodes in the armpit. That combination of findings indicated that there was a fairly high probability that some microscopic deposits of cancer might have planted themselves elsewhere in your body. Don't you remember the analogy of the dandelion (1) on your lawn and its seeds that may travel anywhere and that this is why you received the chemotherapy and why you are still maintained on hormone treatment. If you remember, I had explained that to you both when you first came to see me."

"Yes, I remember," said Mr. K. while his wife shook her head affirmatively.

"Well now it is evident that this suspicion is confirmed and that tumor deposits called metastases have grown in the liver. Again let me emphasize that these are *breast* cancer deposits. They do not represent cancer arising from the liver itself. That would be totally different and far more serious."

"But," she said, "wasn't the chemotherapy supposed to prevent this from happening?"

This was another instance of selective hearing, a situation that I had met so many times before and I that would meet again and again. Although I always emphasized the fact that adjuvant chemotherapy was not a guarantee of cure patients frequently perceived it as such.

"The words 'will' and 'supposed to' are never used in this field of medicine. I certainly did no use them. I never use them. The word to use is 'hope". It was my hope and yours that the chemotherapy would retard and possibly prevent this spread from manifesting itself. It may have indeed retarded its growth but unfortunately it has not prevented it altogether. If chemotherapy were assured to prevent this, breast cancer would be curable one hundred percent. It is not so and here we are. But something can be done to stop this. Now please listen and I will explain to you what these shadows on the liver mean and what I plan to do to try to get them to regress."

"But," she said, "I always heard that once the liver is cancerous there is nothing that can be done."

"Not necessarily so. I will try to explain the situation a little better. Your liver is not diseased. It has become occupied by nests of breast cancer. Treatment will not be directed toward your liver. It will be directed against these unwanted occupants. Treatment will be directed against breast cancer and it would be the same if these deposits had been located in the lung or anywhere else. In someone who has had a cancer of the colon planted in the liver the treatment would be directed against colon cancer tissue and so forth. Do you understand now what we are facing and what the general plan is going to be?"

"Oh yes. Now I understand." She shook her head from side to side. "This all so difficult. I guess I will have to receive chemotherapy again."

"Yes. But that is really still quite manageable."

"Will it be stronger this time? It was not bad the last time. I did not even lose all my hair. Are you going to give me the same medications?"

"A couple will be the same but they will be combined with others that you have not received previously.

"It is a much stronger medicine isn't it?" her husband asked.

"All of the medications used for chemotherapy can be potentially very strong or even lethal," I explained. "That is all a matter of the dose and of how frequently it is given. The most important factor is the effectiveness of the medication against that particular cancer. Each one of the medications works differently and that is why I chose to add additional ones. This way the cancer will be exposed to medications it has not been exposed to before and I hope to catch it by surprise so to speak. At present that combination of chemotherapeutic agents is one of the most effective treatments against breast cancer. It has some side effects different from the others and I will explain them all to you. So far do you follow me?"

"Yes," they both replied.

"OK." I reminded her briefly of the side effects of her previous treatment with which she was already familiar. "The same ones also apply to the new medication. All these as you may recall are easy to control."

"Yes, I know and I really did not have as much trouble last time as I had anticipated. If this is the same I am sure I will tolerate it. I hope I do and I hope it works."

"You may also remember that you will have to drink a large amount of fluid particularly shortly after you receive the injections in order to avoid the irritation of the bladder which may result from the elimination of one of the medications in the urine. You remember that don't you.

"Do I ever. I kept running between the refrigerator and the bathroom all day and all night. Drinking the large amount of water is not hard. It is the getting up at night. I have managed before and will managed again."

"Good. Now for the problems specifically associated with the new combination: You will lose your hair, guaranteed, one hundred percent. This is not a probability; it is a certainty. It will happen quite suddenly about three to four weeks after the first dose. If you still have your wig make sure it is styled the way you want it. I know you did not have to use it last time but this time you will."

"I still have it and I will take it out. I never thought I would have to use it and I was even thinking of donating it. I am glad I kept it."

"One additional problem associated with it is that there is a risk of toxicity to the heart muscle."

"Do you mean that I can have a heart attack?"

"No. What I mean is that the effect of each dose is added to that of the previous one. Beyond a certain amount the total dose accumulated over time may damage and weaken the heart muscle. Because of that it will be necessary to check your heart with a special test which is a scan of your heart that will show how it contracts and that will measure the strength of the contractions. It will be checked periodically as the treatment progresses in order to determine if there has been any change in this that may require a change in the treatment. As a matter of fact, in order to have baseline information, this test will be done before you start the chemotherapy. The other problem is that related to the intravenous administration. This as well as other medications that may have to be administered can be very irritating. If it is injected in the veins of the arm, as were the other medications, it irritates them over time and they get inflamed, painful and scarred. It becomes constantly necessary to find new veins and the smaller they are the more they are likely to get painful, scarred and closed. The real problem arises if it seeps out into the tissues outside the damaged vein. This could be a really very serious problem because it can cause a very severe burn. Because of this risk and because of the need for repeated intravenous injections there is a device that is implanted under the skin that gives immediate access to a large vein in the chest. It is called a venous access port and it consists of a small reservoir the size of a bottle cap connected to a long thin plastic tube. The tube is threaded in a large vein inside the chest, the reservoir is anchored under the skin below the collarbone and the skin is closed over it. It is like having a small cardiac pacemaker in place. You can wet the area, shower and swim without problem. When you have to receive your intravenous injections or when blood has to be drawn all I have to do is to feel for this device under the skin, hold it steady an stick a special needle into it through it plastic rubber top and I have immediate access to a large vein with a large blood flow which prevents it from becoming irritating by the injected medicine. This has of course to be done under sterile conditions but it is both practical and safer than injecting in the arm veins. If you are both in agreement with starting this treatment I will schedule the cardiac tests and the procedure to implant this venous access port. That is a day procedure which does not require you to be hospitalized."

"We both trust your recommendations and will go along with the treatment. That is why we chose to come to you in the first place. How long will I have to keep this device on my chest and will it hurt?"

I said: "There will be of course some mild local pain after the surgery but it usually does not last more than a few days and it is easily controlled with mild pain medications. This device may stay for as long as it is needed, months or even years. This can be decided depending on how you do with the treatment. I must add here that I recommended this treatment because I feel is effective, it is tolerable and it is manageable. Yet I must tell you also that there are a number of alternative regimens each of which may work. Another oncologist may recommend something different but I believe the same new medications will be included in most of the alternative treatment regimens. Some may even prescribe high dose chemotherapy with bone marrow transplantation* or stem cell rescue. You may have heard or read about this. It is an option that, if it is considered, should be done only in the context of an investigational program. If you wish to explore this possibility I will refer you to an oncology group that does it. Thus far the long term results have not been better than those of the standard chemotherapy regimens but the idea behind these trials is good and justifies continued investigation along these lines. This avenue of treatment carries more severe acute toxicity and it has been associated with a small percentage of deaths due to the treatment itself. Until now however it has not been shown to have any definite advantages over the standard chemotherapy regimens."

"I have heard about this," Elaine replied, "and as a matter of fact I know of a woman who went through the bone marrow transplantation and was very sick with it. But finally, a few months after it, she had to have more chemotherapy. No. I want to go along the treatment you have recommended. Just tell me what I have to do now."

"OK. I will schedule the tests and the procedure we have talked about. As soon as they are done, within the next week, your treatment will start. Remember we work on this together. Make sure you keep me informed of any problems that may arise during the treatment. All of us in the office will try to make it as little uncomfortable as possible."

Elaine was again up at the front of the battle, at the receiving end of the chemotherapy. While she kept a straight face, what was she thinking? What was she feeling? What would happen when she got home after this visit and after having received the news of her relapse and of the treatment that would follow? What thoughts? What reactions? The contemplation of things to come, no matter how reassuring I attempted to be, foresaw difficult trials along the course of the journey ahead.

The treatment was scheduled and got on its way. Elaine came regularly and, after a few weeks there was some suggestion that her cancer metastases were starting to regress. She tolerated the chemotherapy without any problems other that the hair loss. I kept encouraging her with my evaluation of her progress or rather I thought I was encouraging her by telling her how well she was enduring her treatment but she did not seem as happy about these good reports as I would have expected. Then, one day, she suddenly started crying as I was examining her. "I guess by now it is obvious that this treatment has failed. There is no point in going on with it, is there?" she managed to say between her sobs. I succeeded in calming her down and asked her why she thought so when I kept telling her that the medications were starting to show their healing effect on the cancer.

"I have almost no side effects," she finally said. "So, I guess it is not working."

I was finally able to explain to her and to convince her of the fact that response to chemotherapy was not a matter of "no pain, no gain" and that her good tolerance of the treatment made it possible for her to receive the optimal and most effective doses of the anti-cancer medications and that this was good, not bad, news. As we talked for a while it turned out that she had been ruminating this misconception for a while and had felt increasingly frustrated and disappointed while continuing a treatment that she was convinced was doing nothing for her. She finally smiled for the first time in a few weeks, with smile of hope.

At about that same period my son and colleague Paul Greenberg was the first to document the lack of additional benefit from that treatment program compared to a standard chemotherapy regimen. This was subsequently confirmed by others.

HERE I CAN CRY CAN'T I?

There is always a box of tissues at hand on my consultation office desk and on the examining room desk. The shedding of tears constitutes an integral and necessary part of cancer treatment and follow-up. It is tension relieving, it is a means of wordless expression of feelings and it is also an occasionally needed method of self-gratification. Gertrude had a great need for the emotional release afforded by the shedding of her tears.

She had come one day for the follow up evaluation of her response to a newly started hormonal treatment. She talked fast as usual, so fast that she had trouble catching her breath, half smiling and half crying, fearing, as always, that she would die soon, seeking reassurance and yet not believing me when I confirmed the fact that she remained healthy in spite of the cancer which had spread into her bones and lymph nodes.

"Excuse me for being so nervous. I cannot help it but please tell me, am I going to die soon?" she asked again on that day as she had at almost every visit for the past several years.

Gertrude was a sweet woman, very nervous, very anxious, tearful and always frightened. She was, however, a person that I could not help but like even when I had to spend a long, unscheduled time to reassure her each time she came. When a "visit" was over, after I had set her next appointment and I finally returned to my consultation room, she would walk meekly into my room and ask again many of the questions I had already answered many times before or even on that same day. She needed more reassurance and even that was not enough.

So each time she asked if she was dying, I would answer: "Of course not. Haven't you looked at yourself in the mirror? Yes, you have cancer, but it is not progressive and you are basically healthy."

"You don't mind if I cry here, do you?" she asked that day with a mixture of a smile and a frown on her tear-streaked face.

"Of course not. I know this is not easy. You are taking all of it with great courage and yes, you are entitled to cry."

"I don't cry at home you know," she then added in a little meek voice. "I don't cry anywhere. I don't talk to anyone about my illness or about my fears. I go about life as usual and no one knows how I feel. I take care of my house, my husband, my children, I help friends whenever I can but here I can cry, can't I? I cannot help it if I am nervous. You don't resent all my questions do you?"

"No I don't and yes you can cry here," I reassured her.

She smiled with tears in her eyes. "You know," she said, "I do all sorts of things for others and every so often when I feel sorry for myself I treat myself to a small shopping spree." Now she really smiled, a nice bright smile on her chubby face. "It's all right to do that isn't it? After all I can afford it and I feel a little better after that."

I told her that this was an old sexist remark that said that when a woman feels bad she should go and buy herself a hat. Whether hats are in fashion or not there is nothing wrong with a little self indulgence, including a piece of chocolate, if it helps one feel better.

"You are very kind and you always make me feel better," she added still with tears in her eyes but a smile on her lips, a gentle and sad smile.

"You are a very nice person," I answered, "and I am glad I can make you feel less sad, but I truly meant what I said: You are really doing well. You are not dying in the sense that the end is about to happen. We are all going to die but right now no one and certainly not you should be counting your days."

"An occasional cry," I tell those who do cry in my office, "is OK. It is good. It helps wash the soul but be careful not to overdo it and drown it."

TWENTY YEARS AND STILL HERE

Sarah was beaming. She came in with a bunch of colorful flowers for our office, a box of cookies for our coffee break and her best smile for me.

"Is this not a beautiful day," she greeted me with as I entered the examining room. "It is a special day, you know of course".

Was I missing something? I looked in the cover of her medical record for her day of birth but today was not her birthday. I must have looked a little puzzled as she smiled at me.

"This is our twentieth anniversary and here I am twenty years later.

Indeed, as I reviewed her clinical summary which is always at the front page of her record I noted that she had undergone her first mastectomy for breast cancer in 1978, her second one for another primary cancer in the remaining breast, in 1980 and then she has later developed metastases, and yet here we were in the year 1998.

How could I have missed this considering that Sarah is on my winners list? That list consists in the names of the women who in my forty years of breast cancer practice had lived more than ten years after they had developed metastases, lived comfortably *with* their cancer. They made up the group of those I called "healthy people with cancer".

"So, are you going to celebrate the day?" I asked.

"Luigi and I are going to celebrate the year. We are leaving for Europe in two weeks for a month. This is something we were waiting for and that I almost never expected to happen after all I went through and thanks to my doctors."

She was so happy and so was I. Sarah had come to consult me for chemotherapy after her first mastectomy. She was treated for a year and then had developed another early cancer in her other breast and underwent her second mastectomy a year and a half after the first one. In 1983, a breast cancer metastasis appeared in her sternum (breast-bone). Since, after a thorough evaluation, it appeared to be the only detectable cancer deposit I recommended that its surgical resection be considered. After his understandably initial resistance to performing this serious operation on a patient with a presumed limited life expectancy the consulting thoracic surgeon eventually agreed to do it. He removed at the same time additional tumor tissue that had penetrated into her chest cavity behind the involved bone. I gave her two more years of chemotherapy after which she remained well for another two years.

Then one day she came in my office very distraught. She had to resign her position as one of the book keepers in the small company where she worked because it had become apparent that for several weeks she had been making errors in her book keeping. She kept missing an entire column of numbers on the right side of the accounting books although in all other ways she was doing quite well. That immediately raised the suspicion a brain lesion and I was not surprised when an MRI study revealed the presence of a lesion in the left side of her brain. It was again a solitary lesion and after a consultation with a neurosurgeon she agreed to undergo a surgical resection of that lesion followed by radiation therapy to the whole brain. She recovered fully and rapidly except for her inability to continue with her accounting work.

When she developed a bone metastasis a few years later hormonal therapy was started in spite of the fact that neither of her two breast cancers had been hormone receptor positive (indicating absence of sensitivity to hormonal treatment) when initially tested and she was still maintained on that treatment. Her bone lesions while still visible on the bone scan had shown definite evidence of healing.

Here we were twenty years after her original breast cancer and fifteen years after her first metastasis, with cancer still present and with Sarah still well in spite of it, carrying on with her life and planning her month in Europe.

Over the years we had inevitably become friends. She had carried her burden with courage and equanimity with the support of her husband Louis, Luigi to all his friends. He came to our office with her most of the time and one could see immediately how close they were. She was one to address any woman waiting to be seen for the first time in our waiting room and reassure her if she felt that person was apprehensive.

I could call on her to infuse some hope into those who were losing it. Her positive attitude was contagious and she was an inspiration for all those who knew her. My wife Anna and I were among the first to be invited to her fiftieth birthday party and she attended all the functions of the charitable foundation we had created to support clinical research projects in the field of cancers of the breast and of the prostate.

"From where I stand you are well," I said after completing her examination. "Enjoy your trip with your husband, send me post cards from wherever you are. You have made my day today. All our patients should be like you. This is indeed a very special day and I wish you many more to come."

"Tell me: Do you think I can be cured considering all the time that has gone by?" she asked.

"I don't know but it does not matter whether you get cured or not as long as you are healthy, to use a euphemism, and as you and your cancer continue to manage to stay together for the next forty years without it hurting you anymore than it is doing now, in peaceful coexistence so to speak. You may know the Jewish saying that goes like this: cancer schmancer, it does not matter as long as you are healthy"

"That is very true."

Before she left the office with her husband she gave me a big hug. That was to be her last.

On the day before she had been scheduled to leave for Europe, I received a message at our office from one of her close friends. Both Sarah and Luigi were killed instantly the night before in a freak car accident in which they were the passengers. We were all devastated by the news. How could this have happened to this particular couple who had struggled so hard for Sarah to stay alive and well against all odds?

How could this happen to *me* after all my efforts to tame the disease that should have killed her a long time ago?

I was overcome with deep sadness and frustration.

Would she eventually have died of her cancer? Was this accident fate's way out for her?

I have faced that question on a few occasions both when a cancer reactivated after many years killing its bearer as well as when such a patient died of unrelated causes after living for years with her cancer. I have no answer. I have followed many for whom I have been able to keep the malignancy quiet for so long that I would sometimes delude myself into believing that this could go on indefinitely, only to find otherwise one day.

Is there such a thing as destiny? I do not rationally think so but in the face of events such as the one that ended Sarah's life along with Luigi's, I allow myself to wonder.

PLEASE NO HEROICS

When is the journey over? Who decides that it is over? What is that decision based on? Can one plan for the end of that journey ahead of the event?

Phyllis Harrison was 75 when she first consulted me for the treatment of breast cancer that had spread to her bones.

She was a spinster who had developed a very successful interior decorating business. She had done it all by herself, was well known and respected in her field and had decorated some of the most famous residences in the United States.

Yet, when she became ill, she was truly alone. Friends and business colleagues visited her, sent her flowers, but she had no one close to give her not just the help that she could manage on her own but the much needed emotional support that is essential in this hard situation.

She was fortunate enough to be able to rent, buy or hire the services she needed, and she did. A level headed businesswoman, she knew her circumstances were such that she could count on no one but herself. She had accumulated the means to make her life comfortable and she used them.

On this day when she first sought my advice and care, she made sure that I understood something else.

When we sat in my consultation room after I had finished taking her medical history and examining her, I spent some time explaining her condition as well as the treatment I recommended. After carefully listening to what I had to say, she expressed her view of her condition:

"I understand all you have told me quite well," she said, "and I am quite willing to give treatment a good try. I do enjoy life and what it offers to me. I like the company of my friends, the visits to the museums, the art shows, the music and all that. However, if treatment does not offer me the possibility to continue to have at least some of that I don't want to go on living simply for the sake of being alive on a day by day basis. I want therefore to make this clear to you from the very start. I want no heroics. When it is time to go I want to be able to go simply and comfortably. After all I am 75 and I have had a good and successful life. I am no longer looking for more of it in terms of quantity. I am looking for quality. I hope this is acceptable to you and that you will agree to care for me under these circumstances."

This was said simply, clearly and deliberately. This lady had obviously thought it through long before her visit to me, even probably long before she had developed breast cancer. Unlike most people, she had not been one to wait for the crisis to make her end of life decisions. Her approach to this appeared to have been the result of a well thought rational evaluation of her condition.

"I have no problem with this," I told her. "My philosophy of treatment is to treat as long as there is treatment available that also offers a reasonable likelihood of causing a regression of the cancer and relief of its symptoms, while also being tolerable. When the expected benefits of such treatment become minimal in terms of their probability of occurrence, quality and duration while its side-effects are anticipated to be increasingly disruptive of the quality of life, I find it quite acceptable to direct and limit patient care to the relief of symptoms for the balance of this life. That is good and appropriate treatment at that stage of the disease. If you chose to have me treat you I will always make sure to explain discuss with you any and all the changes which have to be made from time to time before proceeding with any new treatment."

"That is truly what I had hoped to hear." She had been somewhat reticent during this conversation but now she appeared more relaxed. We were on the same wavelength.

"There are still some things which are advisable for you to do as I undertake to treat you," I added at this time. She waited for me to continue.

"Given what you have told me, it would be advisable for you to prepare and sign some documents instructing me to do just what you told me. One of them is called a living will or advance directive. I will try to find a sample copy for you to use as a model to write your own. You might want to consult your attorney about this before you execute the final document. Another one should state the identity of a surrogate you should designate to make decisions for you and to carry out your instructions in case you become physically unable to do that yourself. You may incorporate that in the previous document but your attorney should advise you about this also."

She told me that her attorney had already had her sign these papers several months previously when she had re-done her will. She had copies of these some place at home.

"That is good but it is very important that I should have a copy of each in your medical record at my office," I told her.

She agreed and promised to mail them to me.

I then told her about another document regarding what she would wish to have done if she suffered an arrest of the function of her heart and lungs.

"You mean when, not if, Doctor. That is for sure going to happen and probably sooner than later. And before you ask me my answer is no." She was very emphatic. "No, I do not want to be resuscitated... for what? No! I plan to die only once thank you, and I want to be assured of that."

"Well then I will prepare this document and keep it in your file. You should also know that whenever you are hospitalized, and each time you are, I will ask you this same question and will enter a similar dated document in your hospital record. In this way you will not find yourself inadvertently hooked on to a mechanical and electronic life support system, unnecessarily and against your wishes. It is better not to initiate a course of action that is expected to be futile because once artificial life support has been started it is very difficult to interrupt it. There should not be any misunderstanding about all this. I am not suggesting that you prepare all these documents because no treatment is anticipated. I wish to assure you that I plan to treat you and make you feel better to the best of my ability. These documents are to be available essentially for use in the situations I have explained to you. I also wish to add that this is usually not an easy conversation to have with anyone. But then, you are not a usual person and I feel I can explain it all to you now that you have already expressed your wishes to me about the care you wish to receive including the procedures you do not wish to undergo at the end of life."

She gave a long sigh.

"You certainly can. I realize now that it is not always easy to die... simply to die, these days," she added with a little sadness.

"Indeed no," I acquiesced, "but it is easier for those who have given it serious thought before the final crisis of their health and life and who have taken the time and made the effort to discuss it with their family, their attorney and their physician." I assured her again of my resolve to keep her as comfortable as I could make it when the end of her illness would be close as well as at any time during the course of any treatment."

Miss Harrison remains one of the very few persons I have known over the years, who have demonstrated such a straightforward approach when faced with such important, and so frequently ignored or deferred, decisions about life and death.

So many times have I had to present this problem to someone who had just been hospitalized for the treatment of her progressive cancer or of a major crisis complicating its course, a person knowing to be very ill and hoping to get better. That is when I come to see her and I am required to ask if she wants to be resuscitated should she die while in hospital. She is here because she wants to live and here I am raising the probability that she might die. As discretely and as delicately as I can explain the reason for this question her perception has to be that there is a possibility that she might die while in the hospital she has entered in order to remain alive. Each time I have to do this in order to prevent finding one day that person subjected to an unwanted and frequently futile terminal therapeutic exercise, I have to stop for a few minutes and brace myself for the possible emotional reaction, for the questions I will have to answer and for my attempts at reassurance.

In our western society the overwhelming majority of individuals will not open such a discussion while they are relatively young and in good health. Very few will react positively and unemotionally when they have to face and answer such questions. I presume that other societies may have different attitudes about this. Religion and faith certainly play an important role in people's attitudes toward life and death since they do address these questions in some ways. Education should somehow cover these topics but ours mostly ignores them. Few are those truly prepared to address these issues except for those who, through either faith, experience or introspection, have contemplated the finality of their life, not morbidly but rationally, periodically, and given its end the attention it truly deserves.

COME TO MY WEDDING

"Come to my wedding," was the greeting I received on entering I entered Kay's room as I made my hospital rounds.

That was a bit of a surprise. The lady was in her early sixties and had been living with her "ex" for quite a while. She was a highly placed executive in a public relations firm she had helped create several years previously and was not the type to make rash decisions in her life. Her ex-husband was a writer.

"You see," she explained, "my husband and I were married for several years. We argued and fought all the time until we felt that our relationship had become untenable. When we finally divorced we calmed down and were able to maintain a very amicable relationship for several years. I then realized slowly that, while I could not live with him, neither could I live without him." She gave a little laugh. "Life alone was too dull. So as we developed greater tolerance between us we got back to living together, in sin," she added with a chuckle, "for the last several years, giving one another enough space such that now we can truly enjoy our mutual company and it has worked very well. I guess we were meant for each other but not in a marital state."

"Then how and why did you decide to get married again?" I asked.

"One thing is that we have little time left with my cancer progressing at an increasing pace during the last few months. This will then make the settlement of any estate I leave when I die, easier to manage if we are again legally married. We have no children and neither of us has any close family. He will be the main beneficiary and I don't want to leave him with any problems. A this point marriage will not change anything to our relationship which is quite happy."

At the time of this conversation, Kay had been hospitalized because she had developed fluid in the pleura, the inner lining of the chest, around her right lung as a result of the progression of her metastatic breast cancer. Out of her chest came a tube, that had been inserted for the purpose of draining the fluid into a special container. This in turn could be connected to the wall suction outlet located near her hospital bed or could be disconnected and carried around by its handle whenever she had to move around. This contraption was to remain in place for a few days until all the fluid was removed and at that time a medication would then be instilled in the pleural space around her right lung in order to dry it up and keep it from filling again.

The wedding date was set. The nurses on the floor had made sure the conference room would be available. They were all invited along with the house staff physicians on that floor and basically anyone who was around that floor and could spare the time on that day.

When I arrived almost every one invited, a total of about ten people including her surgeon and me, were there. The minister arrived a few minutes later and proceeded to marry again Kay and her ex-husband in a very touching ceremony. There were flowers and ribbons even on the IV pole. Everyone was smiling. The groom and bride kissed, the cork popped off a bottle of Champagne and the large cake was cut. They were wishes of health and happiness in spite of the unhappy circumstances.

"I am so happy all went so well," she told me the next day. "I was afraid I would be ill. Now I can rest. I have done the one thing I still wanted very much to do before I die and now it is done."

The will to complete a task, to achieve a goal, to put the final period to an ongoing work or to witness an event is an element that plays a role in the complex mechanism of survival of people with cancer. Planning for the future or for closure is an important part of the life of the cancer-bearing person and I think it does, for a short period, influence the clinical course of that person. Kay had accomplished what she wanted. Now she could relax. She no longer wanted nor needed to struggle to remain alive. She died shortly after that. That story is not unique. The first time I was exposed to a wedding between a young woman dying of leukemia and her healthy and loving fiancé was while I was in my first year of residency. A few years later a man in his fifties married one of my patients who, at the time, was suffering with progressive breast cancer metastases. Others among the patients I have treated over the years have married under the same circumstances. And so, while I have witnessed the sorrow of women who have been abandoned by their husbands or companions when disease struck, my view of human nature remains on the whole positive. Most couples destined to become or to remain united do so even under the most adverse circumstances.

NO BORGIA METHODS

The search for miracle treatments or cures is always on. The communications media help propagate intriguing stories about seemingly miraculous remedies, anecdotal reports of cures when the battle against a deadly illness seemed lost, when hope in the powers of modern medicine has faded. Based on such stories and reports and based on the perceived guarantee of effectiveness, some patients decide to take a short cut to the publicized miracle drugs to the exclusion of the standard therapeutic arsenal because of its acknowledged shortcomings. And that is what I faced one day when Regina came to discuss with me a new course of treatment that I had planned when she had called me because of the worsening symptoms of her cancer. New metastases had appeared in her bones and on her chest wall and when I started to explain the chemotherapy. "Forget it!" she exclaimed. "I will have none of your poisons."

She had been suffering with pain in the ribs and in the back for several weeks, but never called me and only mentioned them at the time of her examination a week previously. By that time her discomfort had become quite severe. X-ray films had revealed the multiple dark spots in the white structure of her bones, producing a honeycomb appearance in some of these structures, the telltale images of cancer having grown in and destroyed the bone tissue in these areas.

"But without treatment this will get worse," I tried to explain. "At least the chemotherapy gives you a chance for improvement and relief." She had already received hormonal therapy and its benefit had eventually come to an end.

"No a chance!" she replied. "I want none of your Borgia methods of treatment, none of the poisons you use. These will do me more harm than good. They will kill my immune system, that's what these drugs do."

I had heard that exasperating argument from other people on several occasions before. Still, I tried not to sound exasperated.

"Tell me then what your intact immune system is doing for you right now. Nothing! Your pain is getting worse. It is certainly not helping you fight your cancer. Please hear me out. Let me help you."

She folded her arms, stuck out her chin and sighed.

"The proof of the proverbial pudding is in the eating," I explained. Chemotherapy and, if necessary, radiation therapy have been shown to be beneficial. They can cause and have caused cancerous lesions to regress. They don't always do it but this happens often enough and may last long enough to make such treatment worthwhile with good relief of the pain."

"I will have no part of radiation either. It is very dangerous," she retorted.

"Give it at least a try. You can always stop if you don't want it after a trial period."

"No way will I subject my body to such treatment. I will go and receive holistic treatment with immunotherapy. For some time I have felt the cancer was active again. I just wanted to let you know of my decision. I am going to a Caribbean island clinic where they treat cancer with natural diet, with boosting the immune system and not with poisons. That is what I want."

That conversation had taken place years before the studies of the body's immune mechanisms had finally led to some understanding of its various components and of their function in the course of cancer growth, and of the still slowly developing applications of these findings to treatment. But "boosting the immune system" was and is a very scientific sounding word that was and still is frequently used during such arguments.

"Oh! I know about it," I told her. I had indeed heard of that clinic that operated outside the regulations of the United States. I tried to explain to her that she would be wasting precious time if she decided to take that treatment alone without any of those I had recommended. "At least," I asked, "have you investigated this before going there? Have you met anyone who has been treated there and improved?"

"I have read a lot about it," she replied, "and I have been very impressed by their reports, and yes, I did talk to a gentleman who was treated there. After his cancer surgery, he was told he had nine months to live if he did not take any chemotherapy. He is alive now two years after having been treated at that clinic and is doing very well." Then jutting her chin forward, she added: "You cannot argue with that!"

I tried to explain the fallacy of that argument, that it is not possible to tell that his survival was the result of the treatment he received at that clinic and not as a result of the good surgery that had been performed. "The trouble with this type of information," I tried to tell her, "is that neither you nor I were present at the conversation this man had with his physician after the surgery. It is likely that after a lot of questioning about how long he might live his physician probably told him that the *average* survival for his particular cancer at that particular stage was nine months. That means that the range could be anywhere from a few weeks to several years but *averaging* nine months. For this one individual this is meaningless. He might very well have lived the same two years or longer without any of the treatment given to him in that Caribbean clinic or anywhere. Those who dispense the treatment at that or other similar clinics have never published any of their results showing that when their treatment is given alone to someone with a progressive cancer it can make the cancer regress. They talk of curing cancer but have not subjected any of their results to objective scrutiny. Then when their treatment fails they tell the patient that she or he came too late or that they should not have had any chemotherapy previously, that they could have been cured if only they had come right away. If this were true, someone there should have received the Nobel Prize for medicine."

Her face was set. "You will, of course, never accept that there is another way to treat cancer," she added as her final statement. "The medical establishment does not want it for obvious reasons. Anyway, I am going there."

She went, and I did not hear from her for a couple of months. When she finally returned to New York, she was in a desperate condition. She still refused any anti-cancer treatment but accepted to be placed in a hospice program in order to be kept comfortable for the balance of her days.

A legitimate oncologist will never promise success for an anticancer treatment. He or she will relate the fact that such a treatment may be effective, mostly temporarily, but only some of the time and that it is only after an adequate trial that it may become possible to determine whether this is happening as hoped.

Because of the limited effectiveness of the available anti cancer treatments many fair-minded and intelligent people yield to the appeal of peculiar changes in lifestyle prescribed along with unusual remedies, some of them mysterious, others pseudo-scientific, often delivered by a healer self-portrayed as an underdog of the medical community, working alone in a laboratory and shunned by the so-called "medical establishment." A few of the claims may eventually turn out to be real but most are not. Sorting them is a quagmire. Those drawn into that therapeutic course, to the exclusion of those measures with a track record of, at least, some effectiveness, may be losing precious time along with the window of opportunity for a possibly effective treatment. Moreover, such untested therapeutic endeavors, almost always very costly, result in a serious financial drain for the patient.

Many medications including some of the most active anticancer ones have been originally extracted from plants. I am sure there is still an entire pharmacopeia derived from plants and trees waiting to be discovered and tested. In some countries many of those herbal medications have been used for centuries with some measure of success. This unfortunately does not mean that they all are effective. Many of them are not and some of them are dangerous. They deserve investigation rather than blind application based on unproven claims. "All that is natural is not necessarily good," I keep telling some of the people who tell me the stories about "natural" remedies by self-proclaimed scientists, adding, "hemlock is natural but it isn't good. See what happened to poor Socrates when he drank it." I had, on one particularly exasperating occasion in the past, used a scatological analogy, but polished my language thereafter.

SECTION III
LIVING

****

Living is unconscious. How many of us are truly aware of our own life? We are aware of our pleasures, our worries, our discomfort, our suffering, our anguish, our anger, our fears, our friends, our acquaintances and enemies, our duties and responsibilities but are we aware of our *life*? We journey through it not truly aware of its existence.

All of a sudden the one who has been told she has breast cancer becomes aware of her life as an entity that had been there all the time but that becomes suddenly recognized because it is suddenly threatened. What is going to happen to this life, which went on, unnoticed until then? Will it go on? Will it stop soon? How and when will the end happen? What about all the other things and the people who populate this life? The plans, the dreams, the relationships, what will happen to all this?

I will not delve into the metaphysics of life, but will relate in this section the attitudes and compromises that make it possible for many and could make it possible for more to continue to live as close to a normal lifestyle as possible under the circumstances of the diagnosis and treatment of breast cancer.

The story of a physician, a pathologist, I treated many years ago illustrates one these attitudes. A long time inveterate smoker, she had finally been diagnosed with an inoperable cancer of the lung. She herself had confirmed her diagnosis and she had come under my care for chemotherapy. She was quite ill, had stopped working and had filed for disability benefits, living in part out that as well as out of the savings and investments she had accumulated during her active years of work. She was an opera and music lover. When finally faced with the eventually fatal connotation of her diagnosis, she accepted her fate and decided to reorganize her life along her personal priorities. At that time, the chemotherapy was administered weekly and for the following two to three days she would remain quietly close to home. At that time most of the relatively new medications we apply nowadays to relieve and prevent the many uncomfortable side effects of the chemotherapy were not available. Starting on the third day she would feel better and would go out with friends every evening for dinner after which she either attended a concert or the performance of an opera. She went on opera trips to Europe. She experienced an unprecedented regression of her lung cancer and thoroughly enjoyed every moment of her remaining life that she could. She enjoyed her trips, her many social activities and the company of her friends.

She lived!

As a matter of fact, she lived so fully that one day, five years after she had first been diagnosed, she told me that if I continued to treat her successfully she would have to return to work because she would not be able to afford this style of life indefinitely. Life being what it is and guided by mysterious forces, one night, just as she returned home from an evening spent at the opera, she died suddenly of a heart attack. She had not known yet that the last x-ray films of her chest taken a couple of days earlier had shown some starting re-growth of the cancer, not enough to constitute an immediate threat to her life but such as to anticipate a rapid progression of her illness from then on.

This woman had not wasted her limited years of life in fear, neither had she run frantically trying to drink all she could and more out of the cup of time she had left. She had recognized the eventually fatal outcome of her illness, had accepted it and had organized her life in the style she had wanted. That is not an easy task but it is one that will confront each and every one of those who do not die suddenly and unexpectedly. Most of us do not recognize this fact and, other than buying life insurance policies, make no contingency plans at the time when there is no urgency for it. Most people do not think about this until the time of the crisis, and that is the worst possible time for it. I believe that this physician whose final years I outlined had very likely thought about her last and fatal illness years before it actually happened. This made it easier for her to make what were for her the right decisions when the time came.

BABY?

Part of the process of life is its perpetuation and that process is most frequently stalled or interrupted when a cancer occurs in the young.

Fran was trying to get back to life, as it should be when she asked: "Do you think it is OK for me to have a baby?"

Fran was thirty-two. She had undergone a mastectomy for breast cancer, had received adjuvant chemotherapy and now a year after she had ended her treatment she was asking about pregnancy. Her menstrual periods that had stopped temporarily during and for a short time after the chemotherapy had finally returned to normal. Now she had shot the question.

She and her husband had planned to have their first child just about the time her breast cancer had appeared. That most important event of their married life, of her life as a woman had had to be postponed. Yet, they had not given up. They had wanted to start raising a family and that particularly important part of their life had been placed on hold for almost a year. Life had already dealt her a bad blow previously when she had been involved in a car accident and had to undergo an emergency surgery for the removal of a ruptured spleen. She had almost died that time. Now Fran and her husband wanted to put all that behind them and wanted to go on with their life as it should have been and raising a family meant for them a return to normalcy.

She apologized for the fact that her husband had not been able to come with her on that day having been called urgently at the airport where he worked in airplane maintenance.

"I am going to give you a very long answer," I said, "because it is the only way I can answer this question: First, it is not common to see a woman wishing to become pregnant after having been treated for breast cancer. There are a number of reports in the medical literature about pregnancy following breast cancer many of which indicate no adverse effects on the course of the cancer. Neither does previous chemotherapy appear to affect the course or outcome of the pregnancy. On the other hand, the administration of estrogenic hormones, and by inference pregnancy with the associated increase in estrogenic hormone levels in the body, can affect adversely the course of breast cancer if it has already spread. This is not the case for you. You present no detectable evidence of any breast cancer deposits anywhere."

"Spread of the cancer in the form of metastases is most likely to appear during the first five years after diagnosis and more particularly during the first two of these five years. This means that if you wish to become pregnant it would be preferable for you to wait a minimum of two years and preferably the full five years after your initial surgery. After that the risk becomes smaller although not non-existent. If you had any children already I would advise you not to become pregnant again, but you don't."

She raised both hands up in a gesture signifying that this had been her unfortunate fate and not her wish as tears appeared in her eyes.

I waited a minute until she regained her composure and continued.

"Since unfortunately you don't have any children I understand your wish but you must also understand that there is a risk, not related to pregnancy but related to the nature of the disease. It is the risk of the pregnancy hormones stimulating some, possibly as yet undetected and totally asymptomatic, metastases and requiring chemotherapy again. This risk diminishes with time but should this occur during pregnancy, although not necessarily as a result of it, and should you require chemotherapy again, that could cause serious problems."

She was listening attentively now having given up trying to take notes.

"What problems?" she asked.

"Chemotherapy given early during early pregnancy may possibly cause abortion or possibly congenital anomalies in the baby".

She was obviously perplexed. Having anticipated a "yes" or "no" answer and finding none she now looked for advice, which is all I could give her. She and her husband made a truly charming couple, appeared very devoted to one another and would make, I felt, excellent and loving parents to many children. I could not help but ponder the circumstances which had made it so difficult for them to exercise their natural rights to parenthood while a multitude of unfortunate children simply stumble into this mixed up world and are destined to a life of neglect and abuse.

"I see," she added, "so what do you think I should do?"

I have always thought and stated that life is made up of risks and compromises. Decisions are reached based only on the degree of risk and the extent of compromises whose consequences one is prepared to live with and deal with as long as one understands them. And I told her so. Advice? What advice could I give her? I could only help her through the process of selection. Secretly, I hoped she would take the risk because it was obvious that a child would fulfill a strong desire for the happiness that would come with it. Professionally I could only help her arrive at an informed decision.

"The best will be for you to think over what I told you and to talk it over with your husband before deciding. It might be best after that for both of you to return and talk to me together. In the interim if either of you has any questions call me. Come to see me together and we will talk some more."

She simply sat here silently for a few seconds, her eyes looking brighter due to the tears which had welled up, her face saddened by the disappointment she was experiencing.

She thanked me for talking to her and added that although she was leaving without having arrived at a decision our conversation had at least helped her think more concretely about her plans for a family. "If you don't mind," she added finally, "I will come again with my husband so that you can repeat to him what you told me and answer some of his questions."

I kept thinking of one of my first patients who had developed her breast cancer at an early age and who subsequently had five children. Although she eventually developed metastases many years later and died years after that due to the progression of her disease, obviously unrelated to her pregnancy, she had experienced the joy of raising a large family in spite of the proverbial sword that had hung over her head for such a long time and that had eventually fallen.

Neither could I help recalling one of the first patients to consult me after I had just started my private practice. She had been a young woman in her mid twenties who had just had a baby. A lump had appeared in her left breast while she was pregnant and was passed as a "milk cyst." It continued to grow throughout the pregnancy. When it was finally diagnosed as breast cancer after her delivery it had already spread extensively in all her bones. Nothing! No treatment whatsoever had altered its course by the slightest degree. It went on relentlessly and she died within two to three weeks after having consulted me, leaving a distraught young husband in charge of taking care of a newborn infant.

Other women have been cured and lived their natural life with their health unaltered by either having exercised their right and desire of motherhood or without it. Fran's future could be only foreseen in terms of statistics or probabilities. Her will as an individual would prevail over all the other considerations.

I did not know what would be Fran's and her husband's decision but I hoped that some time in the not too distant future she would come to see me with a bouncing baby in her arms.

And sure enough she did. She was still doing well many years later at the time of the writing of this book.

HORMONES FOR HEALTH AND BEAUTY

The examination had been completed and it was time for the questions. Sandy was in her late fifties had undergone breast surgery and had received chemotherapy for breast cancer six years earlier. She had no sign of any malignancy and was doing very well.

"Should I be taking any hormones?" she asked still wrapped in her salmon pink paper examining- gown, seated on the edge of the examining table.

This was going to require some discussion and explanations.

"Why don't you get dressed and join me in my office," I told her, "we will talk about it there."

When Sandy walked in my consultation room she looked great in her summer dress and many heads would turn when she walked in the street. She was truly a beautiful, healthy-looking woman, not at all the sickly one the books and movies frequently depict as the chemotherapy-burdened, cancer-afflicted person.

"Why do you want to take any hormones?" I asked.

"Many of my friends tell me I should in order to stay young and beautiful, to protect my bones against osteoporosis and to protect my heart. Also my gynecologist asked me to check with you about taking hormones. He wants to prescribe them but I told him I have to talk to you first. I am, of course, afraid to take any because I had breast cancer but I don't know what to do. What do you think? Should I? Shouldn't I? Will I get old and shriveled if I don't take any hormones?" she added with a smile."

"I will answer your last question first and my answer is no, you will not shrivel like the lady who left Shangri La. When you say hormones you mean of course female hormones, estrogens... I know. The papers are full of articles about the menopause, the aging process, osteoporosis, coronary heart disease, Alzheimer's disease, and how well estrogens can prevent these problems. It is as if these hormones represent the fountain of youth for every woman. One must read these reports very carefully however. Firstly, they address only these problems in the otherwise healthy postmenopausal woman. There is always in the text some mention of the risk this treatment could create for the woman who has had breast cancer not to mention some other potential risks and side effects. These remarks are often overlooked by the reader who is impressed by the benefits... which are also real."

"I know," she replied. "I realize that and that is why I don't know what to do and what to say."

"You are not the average woman and neither are you the only one to raise this question here," I explained. "I am very concerned about prescribing estrogens for the woman who has already had a breast cancer. The articles you mention do not apply to people like you... Let me ask you a few questions and you will understand why. Do you still have bad hot flashes?"

"Not really. I still have some but they are not truly disturbing. Do you remember how bitterly I complained during the chemotherapy and for a few months after it was completed? That was terrible. I could not sleep through the night. I was uncomfortable and self-conscious a work. I would suddenly turn red and sweaty at the oddest time. That was bad. What I have now is nothing comparatively. They don't trouble me much anymore."

"Do you sleep well?"

"Yes, most of the time. I wake up once or twice a night to go to the bathroom but otherwise I sleep well. Thank God I no longer have these terrible sweats at night."

"Do you have any problems with vaginal dryness, burning or difficulty at sexual intercourse?"

"Not now. I had a lot of discomfort towards the end of the chemotherapy but I used a vaginal cream as you had told me at the time and it helped a great deal. I still use it sometimes, but intercourse is OK now. It's even good."

"Do you achieve a climax?"

"For a long time I did not, and neither did I miss it. My husband was unhappy, but he is very good and has been very patient, I must admit. Since the chemotherapy was stopped, things have definitely improved and now at least I am able to enjoy sex most of the time. It is not the same as before, but it is certainly better than it had been for a while."

"Are you feeling depressed at all?"

"Sometimes. After all, the breast surgery, the radiation therapy and the chemotherapy were not exactly a picnic. Then, of course, there is still not a day I don't think at one time or another about the cancer but I am not morbid about it. I have done what I could, you are doing what you can and I am going on with my life."

"Well, you have told me what I need to know before talking to you about estrogen replacement."

"Firstly, estrogens are not the fountain of youth. Yes, they do constitute the best treatment for menopausal symptoms but all menopausal symptoms do not necessarily require treatment. If some do they do not necessarily require estrogens. If estrogens were not associated with some problems and risks associated with breast cancer, there would be no question about their use for menopausal problems in someone like you. Unfortunately, they are not totally innocuous. Other measures may often relieve the most uncomfortable symptoms of menopause. The problem with estrogens and breast cancer is that there is a definite relationship between them. Breast cancer is often influenced in its growth by estrogens: they can frequently stimulate its growth. When this happens, eliminating their major source, the ovaries in pre-menopausal women or blocking their effect with hormone suppressive medications, both in pre- and post-menopausal women, may cause that same breast cancer to regress. While this is not always the case it is the reason why it is still almost universally accepted as axiomatic that estrogens should not be administered to any woman who has suffered with breast cancer. Yet there is absolutely no data showing that the actual administration of estrogens has ever generated breast cancer or caused it to spread. It definitely has been known to stimulate its growth once the cancer is present. On rare occasions such hormonal replacement therapy has been given to women who had previously been operated for breast cancer and had experienced no further problems with that cancer for a long time. No adverse effects related to the cancer were reported but that very small and select group does not constitute a record upon which to formulate any policy regarding the prescribing of these hormones in women with a history of breast cancer. There is simply no reliable large background of information about this question. So, why play with fire unnecessarily?"

"Furthermore," I added, "estrogens do not constitute the unique answer to the prevention of coronary heart disease in the postmenopausal woman and as a matter of fact that benefit is still open to question. Weight, diet, exercise, metabolic problems such as diabetes, blood pressure, stress, and genes all have a very important role there. The great majority of these except for the genes can be managed to a great extent without estrogens in the clinical setting in which estrogens should be avoided. Of course, it is easier to take a pill a day than to diet, exercise, and basically try to control the risk factors by means other than a single medication. I don't mean to say that all medications must be a voided. Not at all. They have to be applied selectively where they are the best effective way to control a health problem without, at the same time, creating an unnecessary hazard and one of the additional hazards it that of an increased risk of blood clotting with its associated complications."

"What about osteoporosis?" she asked. "Aren't estrogens the best way to treat and prevent that problem?"

I explained that osteoporosis is clearly related to the normal decrease in the estrogen level which occurs as woman matures and particularly after the menopause although calcium loss from the bones starts around the age of thirty to thirty five but that gradual loss does not necessarily cause a problem in all menopausal women. "Furthermore," I added, "the administration of estrogens is not the only way to take care of the problem of bone loss. Prevention applied early in life would of course be the best way to manage it but it is frequently too late for the woman who is already postmenopausal. Yet there are measures that may slow down the loss of calcium, that may stabilize the calcium contents of bone and which may even increase it."

She was surprised to learn that such results were indeed possible without estrogens. She had heard about other medications to treat osteoporosis but thought these were not truly effective and worked mostly through some placebo effect.

I then explained that it is possible to improve the calcium contents of bones and that the combination of a calcium supplement in the amount of 1,200 to 1,800 milligrams of calcium per day with vitamin D 400 to 800 units per day and regular exercise constitute an effective component of any treatment program designed to stop the weakening of bone structure. A portion of the daily calcium intake may be obtained from milk products in the diet and the rest as a calcium supplement. Exercise is extremely important. The pull of the muscles on the bones is a natural stimulant to bone formation and exercising for at least thirty minutes three times a week is necessary for this purpose. One of the major benefits of exercise is that, by improving muscle tone and body balance, it decreases the risk of falling, which is the major cause of fractures.

"For those who are have not been exercising previously," I cautioned her, "this should be achieved gradually. If you take the calcium and vitamin D without exercising you might as well pour these supplements directly down the toilet bowl without ingesting them first, if you get what I mean. It is not necessary to join a gym. Exercise can be done at home as well as by means of a brisk half hour walk. That is also good for the heart and should best be combined with a low fat-low cholesterol diet with decreased caloric intake for overweight individuals."

"Dieting is the hardest of all," she complained jokingly. "Regardless of my good resolutions the temptations are always there. Going out, guests, the children, any social gathering, all are invitations to eat …no, to overeat."

"If you make the effort to take the calcium, the vitamin D and to exercise," I told her, "you will have taken a significant step toward controlling your future health and you may even find it easier to abide by your dietary resolutions. It is also advisable to measure the calcium contents of your bones at the start of this regimen by means of the bone densitometry test and to repeat it periodically at about yearly intervals. This will help evaluate your response to the osteoporosis prevention or treatment program."

"Do you mean a bone scan like when you checked me for the breast cancer?"

"No. This is totally different. You had it done almost nine months ago, if you remember."

"Yes that's right, I forgot. But I still don't understand the difference between them."

"They measure different things. The bone scan reflects the biological activity of bone tissue and identifies areas of abnormal activity due to injury, tumor growth, inflammation, etc. Bone densitometry measures the actual amount of calcium in given portions of the skeleton vulnerable to osteoporosis changes. These are mainly the spine and the hips. If there is evidence of some calcium loss but it is not at a potentially dangerous level at which the risk of fracture with relatively modest injury is high, the regimen described above may be adequate to start. If on sequential determinations of bone densitometry, it is found that no further calcium loss has taken place the same treatment can be maintained. If, on the other hand, calcium loss progresses, other medications are available for treatment. One group of such medications is known as the bisphosphonates*. In addition, a hormone, calcitonin, which works specifically on the mechanism of deposition of calcium in the bones may be effective in stabilizing and improving the osteoporosis process. While they may have side effects of their own, neither of these has any potential adverse effect on breast cancer. And so I try as much as possible to avoid prescribing estrogens to women who have had breast cancer in order to apply the important Hippocratic principle of 'do no harm.' Recently, a new drug has been approved for the treatment of osteoporosis. It is an antiestrogen with estrogen-like effect on bone only. Its chemical structure is related to the one that is used to treat breast cancer, and it seems to be a promising medication. Its wide application to the treatment of osteoporosis in women with a history of breast cancer is still insufficient. This question has actually been addressed at cancer meetings and the consensus is that this medication will have to be studied further before determining how valuable or risky it will be in that particular setting."

"Don't misunderstand me. I am not absolutely rigid about this. I have given estrogens to a very small number of women who have had breast cancer and remained free of any further evidence of this disease for many years but who were so deeply affected by the problems of menopause that their quality of life was seriously impaired and that it was not correctable by any other means. In these few cases the potential benefits of estrogen replacement therapy in terms of their quality of life far outweighed the potential risks associated with it. You are certainly not in this category and you should continue with the program I had started you on after completion of the chemotherapy, and that you have probably not followed."

"Well I have taken calcium on and off but truly not regularly. The exercise… well, that has been harder but I will apply myself to it."

"You really should and you will be due for the repeat bone densitometry in three months. So tell me now, did I answer your questions?"

"Yes, and I am glad I have had the opportunity to talk to you about this. I know you explained much of this to me several months ago but at the time I was so anxious and mixed up that I retained very little of it. I did not want to take hormones anyway because I was afraid. Now I am sure I do not want them. I wish to tell you also that you made this discussion very easy for me. Even my gynecologist has not asked or talked that simply, clearly and comfortably, for me, about the sexual problems I have had, and I thank you for it."

She left leaving, like an afterthought, the slightest hint of her perfume in the room.

In recent years the chronic administration of bisphosphonates has been associated with the rare occurrence of bone necrosis in the jaw sometimes related to recent dental work.

WHAT HAVE YOU DONE...

"What have you done to our sex life?" he asked.

We were sitting in this pleasant garden terrace restaurant overlooking the Long Island Sound. It was a an evening at the end of summer, warm enough to be out, cool enough to be comfortable. The gentle splashing sound of an artificial waterfall and the quiet rustle of the leaves in the breeze added to the relaxed feeling I indulged in after a week's work in my oncology practice. I had planned to enjoy that rare evening in the company of my wife and a couple of our close friends.

As we entered the garden I had passed by a table where one of my patients, Emily, her husband and another couple happened to be seated. I stopped by to greet them and went on to our table at the other side of the terrace. Sometime later Mr. Fischer, Emily's husband, came to the table where we were sipping Turkish coffee and enjoying sinfully sweet middle-eastern pastries and asked if he could talk with me for a moment. We moved to an empty table away from the group of friends I was with. He asked how I thought his wife was doing. An odd place and moment for such a question but I told him she was coming along quite well, free of any problems related to her breast cancer and still on adjuvant hormonal treatment.

"How much longer was she going to be on this medication?" he then asked. He seemed a little ill at ease.

"Barring any unforeseen problems, until she will have completed a total of five years," I told him. Then a little hesitantly and in a low tone, he added: "What have you done to our sex life? I cannot touch my wife; she is so uncomfortable when we try to make love... she even bleeds sometimes. I am sure this is due to the medication. It is terrible. Can anything be done?"

Now I understood his hesitancy and apparent uneasiness. I assured him that things could be done and that since his wife had not voiced any complaints about this I would address it myself at the time of her next visit. He was obviously relieved that he had been able to finally bring this problem to my attention. He had always been present whenever Emily came but she had never talked about this and neither had she.

Three weeks later she came in for her regular follow up examination. In the course of the preliminary evaluation of any health problems or new symptoms since her last examination, I asked her about any menopausal symptoms related to her treatment and in particular about hot flashes and any symptoms of vaginal dryness, discomfort, discharge or burning but made no mention of my conversation with her husband. She then proceeded to tell me about the dryness and in particular the pain at sexual intercourse leading to quasi abstinence.

"I can manage without sex, but it is getting hard on my husband. This is a real problem and I don't know what to do?."

"I wish that you had told me about it before because this can be helped. How was it before you started your treatment?" I asked.

"All was fine. We are no youngsters, but we enjoyed sex. Now," she added, "it's a nightmare."

I had mentioned to her the possibility of vaginal dryness as side effect of going through menopause and with the hormone suppressive treatment when she first started on it. "Have you tried using any vaginal creams to offset the dryness?" I asked.

"No," she said, "I did not know what to do and I could not get myself to talk to anyone about it, not even to my gynecologist. But I am so glad we can talk about it now. What can I do?"

"There are several ways to help you with this problem. Inserting some KY jelly in the vagina before intercourse frequently helps. Try that first. Replens, which is a cream you can buy over the counter or a cocoa butter suppository, may all work as well. I will write these down for you. These are all over the counter products. Try any of them for a few weeks. If in spite of all this you are still very uncomfortable at intercourse an estrogenic vaginal cream may well be a good and effective solution."

"...But is this not dangerous since I've had a breast cancer?" she asked.

"There are still a lot of unanswered questions about this. Ordinarily I avoid prescribing estrogens to women who have had breast cancer in the past. Yet, there are situations where such a person's quality of life is so miserable and the risk of potential reactivation of breast cancer so small that the choice between the two evils is clear. In most such cases a relatively small amount of an estrogenic cream solves the major symptom and may be all that is necessary. While there is some systemic absorption of the estrogen that is very small when the amount of cream that is used is the minimum that relieves the vaginal discomfort. Rarely it may become necessary to use a systemic estrogen in pill form in order to control very severe menopausal symptoms. I have prescribed it in rather rare circumstances and in the smallest amount needed to render severe symptoms manageable. These symptoms don't even have to be absolutely and totally resolved. Reasonable relief is truly what most women in your predicament seek."

"What do you think I should do? Should I take estrogens?"

"Why don't you first try one or the other of the vaginal lubricants I told you about? Here are their names on a prescription blank. Try them for a couple of weeks as I told you and let me know what happens. As I said before, we can then decide whether you should use some of the hormonal treatments starting with the estrogenic cream."

"I am still concerned about using an estrogen because of my history."

"There is another hormonal alternative to using an estrogenic cream or medication:. It is a hormonal medication that is frequently used in the treatment of breast cancer in much larger doses and has occasionally been tried in low doses in women with uncomfortable menopausal symptoms with some good success. It is another possible method of relieving your difficult situation. What I am trying to tell you is that there are many ways of helping you but if you want help you must tell me your problem."

"Now that we have already talked about it, I feel less uncomfortable in mentioning it, and thank you for all the information and advice."

Vaginal lubricants were of little help and Emily eventually tried the estrogenic cream in gradually decreasing amounts over a period of a few weeks to the point where using a small amount of it once every two to three weeks was sufficient to achieve comfortable and satisfactory sexual intercourse.

Some women quickly find their own solution to that problem. When asked if she had any problem with vaginal dryness as a result of her cancer treatment, another lady in her mid-forties told me that she did, "but", she said "I will give you a bit of information you may pass along to others with the same problem. One tiny vaginal squirt of skin cream before intercourse has solved it for me."

TIME

———

"How long do I have?" asked Marcia.

That is the classical question one finds in novels and movies featuring a person afflicted with cancer or some other illness considered potentially fatal. And the question is usually answered with a number sealing that person's fate in a finite time box.

Why on that day? She had been under treatment for metastatic breast cancer for almost a month. The metastases had show up two and a half years after her breast surgery, but she had never asked that particular question. The treatment had barely been started.

"What do you mean by how long?" I asked her in turn.

"Just... how long," she repeated in a low voice.

"Do you mean how long you will live?"

"Well... yes."

"I honestly don't know..." I told her, facing her and looking in her eyes. Seeing the look on her face, I added, "Don't misunderstand me. I am not evading your question. I really, truly don't know."

"But I have cancer, and it has spread."

"Yes, but you have had practically no treatment of any kind thus far and there is a lot of it available. Treatment is very likely to cause your cancer to regress. For how long a period of time no one can predict and therefore you should not count your days nor should anyone else. I would be the last one to set a limit to your life be it only in words. No one can do that and no one should."

"Do you mean that the cancer might stop growing and remain just the way it is now?"

"Not only might it remain stable it is also very likely that it will decrease considerably in size and extent. Actually it may become so small sometimes that it might no longer be detectable by any examination X-ray or scan. While this may last sometimes for long periods of time it does not mean that the cancer is cured... gone... never again to return. It means that it has become so small that it cannot be detected by any of the available tests although it is still there. Even when such a good result occurs, sooner or later the cancer will start growing again and at that time a different form of treatment will have to be applied. Fortunately, there are many different effective methods of treatment that can control the growth of breast cancer. We have not yet begun to fight!"

"I never realized that cancer can actually become smaller. You don't know what you have just done for me. I thought that was it! I was preparing to die. At least now I have some hope. Do you think that if the treatment works I could live for ten or fifteen more years?"

"Why do you want to limit yourself to fifteen years?" I replied smiling at her. "Yes, I think it is possible. It can happen. It has happened although it has been the exception rather than the rule...in the past. But we live in the present and we are looking toward the future and who knows what that will bring? How well you will do will of course depend on whether the treatment is effective and that will not be known until it has been given a good trial. It will depend also on newer development in treatment methods in the foreseeable future. You should not forget that the treatment might also be ineffective, in which case the cancer will continue to progress and a different treatment will have to be started. However, let us accentuate the positive. I plan for your treatment to work and you should plan likewise."

WORDS

The key word of that day was "terminal." Like "how long," that word has been used to seal the fate of the patient in a very finite time tunnel. It should be struck from the medical vocabulary. It serves no purpose and, like the genie of the bottle, once released it cannot be stuffed back in it. Yet there it was... released by this sixty-two year old patient who, in all outward appearances, was the picture of health.

"Doctor, am I terminal?" she asked as we were in the process of reviewing the results of her most recent tests and her planned treatment.

"Terminal?" I asked.

"Yes."

"What do you mean by terminal?"

"My surgeon told me my cancer has spread to my bones and he sent me to you for treatment but I want to know if I am terminal."

"Do you know what that word means?" I asked again.

"Yes, it means I am going to die," she answered looking straight at me.

"Have you looked at yourself in the mirror today?" I continued.

"Why, yes."

We then proceeded with a quick questions and answers sequence.

"And did you find that you looked any different than usual?" I asked her.

"No."

"Do you sleep well?"

"Yes."

"Is your appetite good?"

"Yes, very good alas."

"Do you have any pain?"

"None at all."

"Are you short of breath or do you cough?"

"No."

"Do you do all the things you are accustomed to do?"

"Yes."

"In other words, you are telling me that you feel quite well and, that except for the fact that you will have to receive some medications for treatment, life is proceeding as usual."

"Yes. I guess you could say that, but I do have cancer all over my bones."

"Yes, indeed, and therefore my diagnosis at this time is that your are what I call a healthy person with cancer! Not only that but you haven't even had any treatment yet and there is a lot of it available that can keep the cancer from causing you problems for long periods of time. Now is the best time to start before you are aware that it is progressing and before it starts causing symptoms."

"Then I am not terminal?"

"Not by any stretch of the imagination. Terminal means that not only you are in the last stages of cancer, but also that you have received all possible available forms of effective treatment and that there are none available any longer that would be associated with a reasonable likelihood of improving your condition as well as your quality of life. All that could be done at that particular stage would be to keep you comfortable for the balance of your days. You are nowhere near that stage. Your quality of life is excellent and my purpose is to keep you that way for as long as I can, indefinitely if possible. No, you are not terminal!"

The words and sentences we hear, both grammatical and penal!

"She has six months to live."

"My doctor *gave* me one year."

"He is living on borrowed time."

"What a pity she won't live to see her children grow."

"There is nothing more to do."

"He was told to put his affairs in order."

"Her treatment is in the hands of God now."

"She is terminal!"

All the phrases and statements remembered from the novels, the shows, the books, the stories, the news, the friends, the relatives, the physicians. What power is held by such words and what psychological and even physical consequences they carry! Reality with its incertitudes is preferable to this type of negative power. At least it leaves room for hope.

I WISH

Conversations like the following one make me feel sometimes like the magician at the bottom of the wishing well.

"I wish I could last until my daughter's wedding. I would so like to see her dressed as a bride, be with her, to celebrate with our family and friends..."

"Why should you not be there?" I told Alison.

"It's in fall, nine months from now. That is all I want. After that I don't care."

"Why do you want to limit your life to nine months?" I asked.

Alison remained silent for a moment and she added, "I would so like to see my son graduate from college..."

"I also wish I could live until my grandchild is born. Do you think I will ever see my grandchild, feel small arms around my neck, hear the words I love you grandma?"

So many wishes. So many goals to be achieved with others to follow when the first ones are reached. All to delay the final outcome of that illness.

"Plan to be there. Plan to see what you wish. Without plans you die prematurely in spirit, you die before your time," I told her. I keep telling patients that plans are an integral part of life. They have to be made even if they eventually have to be changed or even cancelled. One must keep planning. "You are still here," I added. "Plan to stick around. I plan to take care of you for a long time."

THE CHOICE

I had just finished explaining the need, the type, the potential benefits and limitations as well as the side effects and risks of the chemotherapy. Grace had developed evidence of spread of her breast cancer in her bones and lungs and had come to consult me for a third opinion about treatment. Both she and her husband had listened very attentively and silently. She had sat there with her hands folded in her lap. He had placed one hand over them. They had remained almost motionless throughout my explanations. She was in her middle forties and he in his early fifties. They were well informed, had consulted other oncologists and had read a lot about breast cancer treatment during the past days as I could judge from the very pertinent questions they had asked me, during the course of my taking her medical history. When I had finished talking they both remained quiet for a while. Then she broke the silence with one question.

"What if I do nothing?"

"Do you mean what if you took no treatment at all?"

"Yes", she answered simply and deliberately.

"What do you think will happen?"

She thought for a moment and then, "I don't know," she said. "You tell me."

"Do you think you will just die?"

She looked down at the floor. "Well... yes...I guess so...I think."

"No you won't. At least not immediately or that easily. Without treatment the cancer will go only one way, worse," I explained. "May be not right away but in time."

"Well, yes. I expect it will and then I will die. And that will be that," she added, now looking at me.

"It is unfortunately not quite as simple because as a result of the progression of the cancer you will eventually become increasingly uncomfortable. You will then ask me or one of my colleagues to help you obtain relief from your discomfort. No pain reliever is as effective as treatment of the condition causing the pain in the first place so why wait until you become so uncomfortable."

"For how long can this go on?" she asked.

"It can be longer than you may think. Much longer. What I am proposing is to try to reverse the course of your cancer now, while it is causing little trouble, in the hope of delaying worse discomfort as long as possible or indefinitely if I can. If without any treatment one would just turn, face the wall and die without any suffering no one would ever go to consult a physician. The main reason for seeking medical treatment is to relieve or minimize suffering. That is why I, as well as my other colleagues you have consulted already, have recommended a course of treatment for you."

"But is chemotherapy not worse? From what I hear and read dying of cancer may still be a better and faster way out."

"Where in heavens do you get all that information? Indeed chemotherapy is neither innocuous nor without its own side-effects but these can be minimized to a very bearable level, and furthermore if, as we all hope, it causes the cancer and its symptoms to regress you will feel much better in the balance. There is a good likelihood that this will happen. There are forms of chemotherapy that are very difficult to take, but with the type you will receive for the treatment of breast cancer you can truly carry on with you life almost as usual. You can go on working if you feel up to it and most people do. You should be able to continue to take care of your household as you have until now," adding "unless you want me to tell your husband that from now on he should start doing the cooking and the laundry."

She smiled for the first time since she had entered the office.

"No," she said, "Gino is really very helpful but I might take you up on it and get a chance to put my feet up once in a while. Truly, I would prefer to have ten times the housework I have rather than have to face what I am... what we both are facing now. I did not know that one could really feel OK while receiving chemotherapy. All the information we gathered about the effects of the drugs is frightening. I was... I am very scared of this whole thing and I had to ask and hear the answer." Then with a sigh she added, "Why did all this have to happen to me?"

"No one has the answer to that but still this problem is manageable. I don't give up easily because I see the good results that come with the treatment, and you should not give up either. I will help you through this whole thing as you call it and let us anticipate success. Unfortunately, the books and articles you read for information about the treatment tell you a lot about the medications, about the cancer itself, but they tell very little about the people themselves, how they manage and what happens to them as persons. So, if you have any questions don't hesitate to ask me."

"We almost did not come to see you today," her husband said at that point, "but Dr. Giordano, our family physician whom you know, insisted that we have this final consultation and I am glad he did."

Gino and Grace Finelli then told me how the two previous oncology consultations had gone. One of the oncologists explained that the cancer had spread and recommended a course of chemotherapy, that he explained, could control the growth of the disease for about a year. He had briefly listed the side effects of the treatment he had proposed and given them a pamphlet to read about it. They were to call him with their decision about starting the treatment. The other consultation had taken place in a hospital setting where she was initially interviewed by a nurse practitioner who took a detailed medical history. She was then examined by a physician in training, a Fellow, who then presented her case to the attending physician she was consulting. She was offered several treatment options as well as the opportunity to participate in an investigational therapy program. They were again given a fairly thick typewritten information document to read about the various recommended treatments and a recommendation to call back with their choice and decision.

"You have given us the same information but with a totally different and understandable perspective on the treatment and we thank you for it," said Gino. "I think Grace will agree with me about going ahead with the treatment."

Grace nodded her consent. "How soon should I start?" she asked.

"Frankly, as soon as possible. There is no true emergency at this point but still it should start during the course of the next few days. You must also decide where you want to be treated since you have consulted three oncologists by now."

"I think Grace agrees with me," he added looking at her as she nodded her approval, "about receiving it in your office. We will make the appointments with your secretary I presume."

"Yes, I will tell her to have you start at the beginning of the week. Again I want to remind you to call me if you have any questions now or during the treatment. I would rather handle small problem early rather than wait for them to become big ones. So, don't hesitate to call."

I cannot feel the anguish of people like Grace and Gino. I can understand it. I feel their need for information in a situation in which Grace's life is literally at stake. I can feel the frustration at receiving a statement, a recitation, a list of the treatment medications, their method of administration, their side effects and other problems, without a conversation about how this was all going to impact upon their life, their day-to-day life, their future, their plans, without at least being offered the opportunity to talk about these. It has to be their choice but that choice must be made in the context of their whole life's structure.

THIS IS NEW YORK

Joan O. was in her early thirties, was divorced and lived with her lovely daughter of 10. Her child was taken care of by her mother while she was at work. She held two jobs, one as an executive secretary in a small advertising company, the other, a freelance work as a "voice" for television ads. She has a young girl's voice that was sought after for certain types of advertisement.

The progression of her breast cancer had necessitated the administration of several months of intensive chemotherapy as a result of which she had become totally bald. There was not a hair on her scalp, but she had a rather nicely shaped perfectly oval head and had decided she did not want to wear a wig.

Whenever she sat, totally bald, in my waiting room, quietly reading a magazine before being called in for her examination and treatment, all the other women sitting there would avoid looking at her. Some even told me how upsetting her baldness was to those who were just starting their chemotherapy.

"It is *her* thing," I would say. "She has accepted her condition and lives with it the way she wants. There is not much I can do about it, and I don't think I should do anything. It is her privilege to appear just the way she is. She is telling the world that the important thing is being here, being alive and feeling well and not simply the appearance of it."

This went on.

One Monday morning when she came to see me she said: "Something interesting happened to me this past Saturday night. It was my birthday."

"Hey, happy birthday. Did you do anything special?" I asked, sensing that she was dying to tell me.

"Thank you and yes as a matter of fact. That is what I wanted to tell you. A group of my friends decided to make a big 'shindig' for my birthday. They reserved a large table at the Tavern on the Green in Central Park, ... in the Crystal Room no less! So, I arrived there at eight o'clock, all dressed up and bejeweled. The place was packed as you can imagine on a Saturday night in this season in New York. It was beautiful! With all the crystal chandeliers and all the people fashionably dressed and all that. Our table was all the way at the end, a choice place near one of the large windows overlooking the park. Of course I wore nothing on my head except my skin."

She chuckled.

"I walked across the entire room to reach my friends already seated at the table. Would you believe that no one along the way or anywhere, not a single person turned around or even glanced at me? No one appeared curious or surprised. No one seemed even to notice me. This is New York!"

Indeed! And Joan was who she was and showed it to the world.

PLANS

Estelle appeared hesitant about something.

"I have a question for you," she finally said.

"Go ahead, ask. I will try to answer if I can."

She and her husband had run their dry goods business by themselves for many years. It had grown and prospered over the years and now their two sons had assumed most of the responsibility for the store. When she had to have her breast surgery and her chemotherapy she retired and her husband Nathan came increasingly less frequently into their business office in order to help her and to drive her to all the various medical appointments and treatments she had to undergo. She was well for the following three years and with the business in the hands of their children they had hoped to start catching up with some of the good things in life that they had missed. Then metastases had appeared and a different treatment had to be started again. Fortunately, she was responding well. Her pain had improved and her x-rays had shown evidence of healing of the metastatic lesions.

"My husband and I never had any real vacation in our entire life," she told me. "With one thing or another, our children and our elderly parents, we could never really take off. This year, however, we made reservations to fly to Europe and travel there for a while."

"Good for you."

"Our reservations are for July this year, in seven months..."

"Well?"

"Well, what do you think?" she then asked. "Should we cancel our plans?"

"Why should you?"

"You know," she added hesitantly... "With the cancer and all that, ... I don't know."

"What do you mean?" I knew what she meant. I just wanted to hear her say it.

She hesitated again and added, "after all, I have cancer and I might... you know."

I had to help her formulate her thoughts. "Do you mean you think you will be terribly sick with the treatment or die soon?" I asked.

She seemed somewhat relieved by my open acknowledgement of her fears. "Well yes! It is possible and even likely isn't it?"

"First," I reassured her, "you will not get awfully sick with the treatment you are receiving regardless of what is shown in all the movies about cancer patients. Nowadays most of the chemotherapy side effects can be prevented or relieved."

"Second," I added, "I don't know when you are going to die. You have an advanced cancer but you are generally well, you have just started your treatment and you have already shown an early response to it. It would be a pity to cancel a nice vacation unnecessarily. If you somehow get very sick and you cannot travel, your trip can be cancelled then. Finally, assuming the very worst, although I really, truly, do not anticipate it at all, and that you do die before July, your trip will really no longer be your problem. Your husband will be the one who will have to deal with the travel reservations, and he will. So, why should you worry about this now?"

"You know, you're right!" she exclaimed, smiling. "You have a good way of downsizing the problems we patients bring to you."

"I plan to get you well and to keep you well. You, on the other hand, should plan to have fun. Think positive."

LOOKING FORWARD

"Mens agitat mollem," or the mind moves the matter. This is what I was taught in high school, and indeed it does when a goal has been set and has to be achieved.

In the short life of Alicia that goal was to be a piano recital she had been preparing for. Alicia was a young concert pianist. She was not well known, she was not a name one would recognize in the music world but music was her life. She had studied, practiced and prepared. She had given a few recitals here and there and had hoped for one in New York. Then the pains started and got worse until it was discovered that these pains were due to disseminated bone metastases from a breast cancer she did not even suspect she had.

At that time, the hormonal medications designed to suppress the production or block the formation of estrogens, had not yet been synthesized. The standard treatment for a young woman at that advanced stage of breast cancer was the surgical removal of both her ovaries. The surgery was eventually performed and her pains resolved almost immediately. Then, over the period of weeks which followed her bones started to heal, she was able to move comfortably almost as well as prior to the onset of her symptoms. She went back to practicing her piano and with the help of her husband started to organize her recital. They chose an all Chopin program, reserved the hall, printed the announcements mailed the programs and invitations, and she practiced and practiced.

"I know I am getting well," she told me at the time of one of her follow up visits at my office, "because I am playing better than I have ever played. I am so looking forward to this recital I can hardly wait."

She was full of energy and enthusiasm.

I was not able to attend the concert for reasons that I cannot remember, although I had planned to and had been looking forward to it almost as much as she had. It went very well. The following week she related to me that the school hall they had rented had been sold out. The audience had clapped her for three encores and she was exhausted but walking on air. The local paper had printed a nice enough review of the event, and when she came to my office she brought me a large reel-to-reel tape of the entire performance. I listened to it from time to time on the old reel-to-reel player I still own. I can still picture her in my mind when I listen to it.

At the time of that visit immediately following her concert, she complained of some aches here and there that she blamed on the physical effort of the performance and the stress of the whole preparation. Her discomfort continued to progress over a short period of time and it soon became obvious that the cancer has started again to pick up momentum.

I believe it is more than coincidental that she was able to proceed with all that it took to reach the goal she had set for herself, the concert. I believe that her mind directed the cancer to stop growing long enough to allow her to reach the day of her planned performance and long enough for her to go through that performance. Once that was done she finally relaxed and her illness took over and took her away in a very short time.

I have not listened to her tape in some time. But, I still do think of her sometimes when I hear a Chopin piano étude or sonata.

TO LIVE, TO LOVE

Four years had passed since Concepción had undergone a right mastectomy for breast cancer. She came originally from Ecuador where she worked for a relief organization connected with a group of North American physicians who traveled in the South American continent at a few months intervals to deliver medical care in clinics located in underserved areas.

She came from what we would consider here an upper-middle-class segment of our population, but was considered affluent there. She spoke Spanish, Portuguese, English and German. Her work absorbed her completely, and while she had at various times been more or less "romantically" involved, she had not found the companion who could share her life without limiting her work and who would at the same time be her intellectual equal. She was a very unusual person; truly dedicated to the poor people she served, extremely bright but without the opportunities to share her intellectual talents with her administrative co-workers.

Whenever she came to New York for her check-up approximately twice a year we would manage a bit of conversation about her work, the drudgery of the administrative constraints and the politicking in the area of the world where she lived and worked, the misery she encountered all the time and about which she could do little more than the organization's work as well as the occasional scary encounters with belligerent groups scattered around the countryside of South America. Above all, she lived in constant fear of breast cancer recurrence in spite of my assurances that the type and size of the cancer she had undergone surgery for, were associated with a very high probability of permanent cure.

I gathered that in spite of a very active life that included a lot of traveling with various groups of both professional and administrative co-workers, she remained somewhat lonely.

On that particular day, four years after her mastectomy, after she had answered my questions about her health status, she finally acknowledged her past fears but also informed me of the fact that she had finally overcome her concerns about her cancer.

"I finally believe you," she said in her Spanish accented English. "I truly believe now that my cancer is gone for good. I feel well, I have no fear and now I want to live, I want to love, I want to go on into the future, I want to have some joy for myself for a change. It is time."

"Well, finally you heard me and I am happy for you. So what does this all mean?" I asked. "What are you going to do?"

"I have requested a prolonged leave. I will visit my family in Quito, travel in the U.S. and in Europe possibly look for a different job, possibly in the government or even better, with an international organization. I don't know. I am keeping my options open. All I want now is to be separated from what I have been doing for years, re-evaluate my life then decide what to do. I have dropped the fear of my cancer. Unloading that was a great step and a great relief. Now I want to take time to look forward. Life is very important. I don't want to waste it."

Concepción is one of many women who while they are truly cured have a hard time believing it. Once this realization is accepted it is as if a new life starts. There is life before the cancer, and then, for these women, follows a period in between, a period which may be described as a dormancy characterized by a form of automatic behavior akin to somnambulism from which they eventually wake up. That awakening is a rebirth, a new life with an entirely new perspective and appreciation of all things. Concepción had just gone through that awakening.

SECTION IV
ATTITUDES AND REACTIONS

****

Over the years during which I have interacted with the people who have come to see me for a medical opinion, for advice and frequently for prolonged treatment I have observed the fact that attitudes have a major influence on their quality of life. As a matter of fact, I have seen the advent of "quality of life" as one of the parameter used in treatment evaluation.

Attitudes have many aspects, that include that of a patient toward his or her illness, the attitude of the treating physician toward both the illness and the patient and the reciprocal attitudes of the patient with his or her personal and professional relations.

While the attitude of the physician is certainly very important, the one that has the greatest influence on the quality of life is the attitude of the person or persons closest to the patient and in particular that of the spouse or of the one now called the "significant other."

The caring and loving support of a spouse or close companion appears to help decrease the intensity of the side effects of the chemotherapy, it relieves the anxiety portion of the pain and other suffering, enhances the positive feelings, increases the sense of security and, in the cases in which life approaches its end, that end arrives through a more peaceful process than when such a support is lacking or when discord has been present.

The attitude of the physician has to be one of realistic optimism. Let us face it, if an oncologist cannot be optimistic, truly deep-down-in-the-heart optimistic, how can he or she give the patient one of the most important ingredients of care that is *hope*. If the physician does not convey the feeling that there is a real possibility of improvement or recovery how can the cancer patient be hopeful of it? I have met a number of people who, at the time of their consultation with me for a second opinion, have told me how reassuring it was to talk to me after a previous experience during which the consultant inferred that while treatment would certainly be recommended it was understood that in the long run it would make no difference since there was no cure once the cancer had spread.

In our present state of knowledge it is very rare for the treatment of cancer in its advanced stages to effect a cure. In the case of breast cancer, however, such treatment is very likely to cause a regression of the cancer for periods that can frequently be measured in months and often enough even in years. During this time other methods of treatment will constantly be developed, as they have periodically been in the past and will frequently be in the future. They will be capable of prolonging the periods of respite from the cancer. Even at these advanced stages, cures have been reported and in my own experience I have observed periods of regression and stabilization of the malignant process lasting more than ten years with good quality of life in many patients. I have reason to be an optimist and I make sure to convey this feeling to those who chose to come under my care.

I have also learned from patients the problems they encounter in their relationships with those around them, how these have affected them and what techniques they have used to resolve them. It is not uncommon for people to avoid contacts with friends or acquaintances who have a cancer because they don't know what to say, what to do, or what attitude to assume. As a result, social contacts have been curtailed and the person with cancer becomes isolated. Consequently, it is frequently the one who is ill who has to help the others understand that illness has not changed their relationship and who encourages them to pick up the relationship where it has been left. In summary, attitude is a frame of mind that can profoundly affect the very fabric of the life of someone who is ill. Inappropriate attitudes, while not always easily perceived, can be recognized and should be modified.

I will always remember a woman in her sixties who was referred to me for treatment of metastatic breast cancer and whose daughter had forgotten to bring with her the letter of reference from her physician. We had discussed her diagnosis and treatment in a very constructive way and she was ready to start as soon as the preliminary tests had been completed in the hospital. While she was appropriately concerned about her illness, her attitude was that I would try my best, she would do likewise and that through that cooperative effort she should contemplate an improvement. She felt positive about the whole thing. However, when I came to see her in her hospital room later on that day I found her totally distraught. Her daughter who had been present at our earlier interview had rushed back to their hotel, had found the sealed referral letter her physician had addressed to me, and had brought it back to her. While her daughter was out of the room for a moment, she had opened it. Upon reading it, she had come across a sentence that stated in essence that this referring physician thought "it was sad that this unfortunate woman with metastatic breast cancer was going to suffer terribly and die soon as a result of her rapidly advancing cancer despite all available treatment."

I was never able to undo the devastating effect this statement had had on her.

I learned early in my medical career the power of words, be they written or spoken, and to weigh carefully any statement I would write or proffer. Many years ago I came across a motto that stated: "Think twice before you speak… then first talk to yourself." This could be said also about the written words.

ANGER

"Let him suffer too," she uttered.

I was taken aback.

This brief conversation had taken place at a time when, after six years of post-graduate training I had, for two years, been in the private practice of oncology with a major emphasis in the treatment of the advanced stages of breast cancer. Lucille K.'s husband had called me from Virginia to tell me that his wife was afflicted with metastatic breast cancer and that he had been referred to me because of my expertise in that field, by a colleague who had trained with me. He had introduced himself, had explained to me how he had come about to call me and asked me if I would accept to take care of his wife. He wanted her to be treated at the Memorial Hospital for Cancer and Allied Diseases now known as the Memorial Sloan-Kettering Cancer Center. He asked me if I could arrange for her direct hospitalization under my care. She was very ill and would have to be flown in by private ambulance plane accompanied by her private physician.

Two days later she was admitted to a large corner room on the tenth floor of the hospital. In the early sixties, there were still different categories of accommodations at our hospital, ranging from large single rooms to wards containing eight to ten beds and up to between twenty and thirty at municipal institutions. Needless to say, the tenth floor had large single rooms that, in addition to the hospital bed, contained a couple of comfortable armchairs and a sofa. The food was of a better selection and, if allowed by the patient's physician, wine could be served with lunch or dinner. Visiting hours were longer. Visitors could order a good meal from the hospital's kitchen. The view out of most of these rooms' windows was great, overlooking the East River and towering over this section of the Upper East Side of Manhattan. One could see some of the river traffic on one side and the city's skyscrapers on the other.

Lucille K.'s treatment was started after the preliminary tests had been completed. Her husband remained with her at all times for the first four days. He left after dinner to rest a little at his hotel and returned an hour to an hour and a half later remaining frequently until she fell asleep late at night. She was in pain and had to receive analgesic medications quite regularly throughout the day and the night. Still she remained uncomfortable. She was not improving.

One morning, as I came out of her room after having examined her and checked on her treatment, her husband stopped me outside her door. He told me he was exhausted as result of the hours he had been keeping and her demands for him to be around at all times. He asked me to suggest to her that since her treatment would go on for several more days he should go back to his hotel to rest for a few hours daily.

I came back in the afternoon to check her condition. She laid in bed with the window shades down and the room in semi darkness. In the penumbra I could see that her eyes were closed. She was not sleeping and she greeted me briefly when I came in. I sat by the side of her bed for a while trying to have a conversation about how she was feeling and attempting to give her an opportunity to talk to me about herself, her life, her illness. I wanted to assure her that I would do my best to make her better and to keep her comfortable throughout the treatment period. After all, I had not known her previously and I understood that the circumstances that brought her under my care were somewhat complex. I wanted to find a way to communicate with her other than that limited to checking her laboratory tests, examining her and giving her my daily professional assessment of her physical condition and of her illness. She was totally unreceptive. Her answers to my questions were laconic and her conversation would immediately drift back to her personal discomfort.

She must have been a beautiful woman when in good health. She was tall, with slightly wavy ash blond hair and had classical regular facial features. Even the scowl, permanently etched on her face, was absolutely symmetrical, from the deep vertical furrow between her perfectly arched eyebrows to those that had formed between her nose and the corners of her mouth. She never smiled. She received enough analgesics to relieve the severity of her pain and yet her bitter expression never relaxed even while she was asleep. She must have been terribly unhappy but I had been unable to have her express any of her feelings. I had finally told her that I had noted that her husband appeared very tired and I suggested to her that she should advise him to retire earlier and have some rest at his hotel. It was then that she communicated to me her feelings, in three short angry words: "Let him suffer," she said. "I am in pain. Let him suffer too."

I had not known these people for more than a few days but could not help feeling quite shaken by this simple statement, which revealed the deep anger separating them already in life before the fast approaching ultimate separation, which would conclude Lucille's fatal illness.

I had been trained to treat *illness*. Understanding and treating *people* had been a relatively neglected part of the medical school curriculum and of the long subsequent postgraduate training during residency and fellowship. Yes, we had received some rudiments of education in psychiatry but young physicians were too busy taking care of a large load of patients for the first part of this training and then taking care of the very sick cancer patients during the second part while at the same time learning the newly developing treatments of this group of diseases, attending conferences and participating in various research programs frequently to the detriment of our own family life.

Lucille's reaction to my question became an important event in a lifelong learning experience in which the women and men who came under my care, also in a way, became my teachers. I never found out the underlying dynamics of the terribly unhappy relationship between Lucille K. and her husband. All I had seen was the profound anger expressed by a dying woman, anger at her husband, at her illness and at a life she was not prepared to leave. I felt that the suffering resulting from this combination of anger and frustration had been as destructive or even more so than her cancer and I doubt that any attempts had been made earlier to recognize let alone address the emotional upheaval which had shattered this couple's life.

This experience was one of many which led me to listen very carefully to the frequently subliminal information and messages passed on to me during conversations with those who sought my advice and treatment.

TIMING

December 23. The end of the year is upon us. So is a long-awaited, brief vacation squeezed in between Christmas Day and New Year's Day.

The most stressful days for me are those just preceding a vacation away from New York. More stressful even are the last few hours before going away. I am leaving in the morning and I am working around the clock until then. All the crises and urgent medical problems presented by the patients must be dealt with and there are always more of them just before a major holiday. All the letters I usually write when I catch up on my work during the weekends must be done before I leave. Telephone calls, that could have been returned in the morning, must be returned now. All the patients' test reports I received over the previous forty-eight hours must be reviewed and many times some treatment decisions must be made based upon these reports before I leave for several days.

And so on that Friday, December 23rd at 9:15 PM, I came across the x-ray films and report of Judith R. She had recently complained of increasing pain in her right knee and the films I was looking at showed that a large tumor lesion, a breast cancer metastasis, had grown in the bone of her right thigh. It had bored a large hole in it, a destructive process that had considerably reduced the mechanical resistance of that bone, raising the danger of fracture with minimal trauma or stress. I was going to be absent for ten days but had to tell Judith to make an appointment with the radiation oncologist to schedule a course of radiation therapy to this damaged part of her bone in order to prevent a possible fracture. I had to tell her to minimize any weight bearing on that leg until there was some evidence of healing of the bone.

She picked up on the third ring and sounded surprised when I identified myself.

"What on earth are you doing working so late? I thought you had already left for your holiday."

"That is not until tomorrow morning," I told her. "I am just clearing a few things before leaving, checking the latest reports and calling people. I am calling because I received you latest x-ray films today and I was looking at them."

"Is there a problem with my knee?"

"Well, yes but the problem is not with your knee. It is with the femur on that side, the big thighbone. There is some damage to its upper part, the part that fits in the hip joint."

There was a brief silence. I hate to give such new on the telephone but I had no choice.

"Are you telling me there in cancer in there?" she finally asked.

Judith was special person, one for whom one feels immediate empathy. She smiled even under adverse circumstances and she had certainly gone through some in the course of her illness. She had become tired of the whole process of repeated treatment and relapses. She needed a rest. I so wanted her to remain well longer but there it was, that big hole where the cancer had grown in her bone. A knot tightened in my stomach.

"Unfortunately yes. There is a deposit of cancer in that part and that is why you had pain in your knee. Damage in the vicinity of the hip frequently causes pain in the knee. The bone has been seriously damaged there and you should receive radiation therapy to that region. I am sending a letter to Dr. Ramsey who treated your breast a few years ago, asking him to start you on a course of radiation to the femur bone as soon as feasible."

"Can it wait? Is it all right to start after New Year?" The knot in my stomach was getting tighter. I longed to be on a beach contemplating the ocean and watching the pelicans dive into it for their meal.

"Yes, since that is only one week away, but call first thing on Monday at least to reserve the time at his radiation unit. That bone is very fragile and may fracture with a relatively minor injury. That is why it has to be taken care of as soon as possible. I also want you to use a cane for support and be very careful not to fall or even to stumble. It *might* be necessary to operate in order to strengthen the bone but with good care you may well avoid surgery."

I was drenched in perspiration.

We talked for a few minutes longer and she promised to call for her appointment.

Ten days later I was back at the office. She came for a follow up examination a couple of days later.

I asked her to come in my consultation room where we could talk a little about the next systemic treatment course. After she settled in the armchair, she started talking.

"Could you not have waited?" she asked. "Could you not have waited until after Christmas and let me celebrate peacefully instead of worrying during the holidays?"

She had truly taken me by surprise.

"I did not think it would have been safe to procrastinate and run the chance of you breaking this bone."

"Would seven or ten days have made so much of a difference?"

Would it? I don't know. I had spoiled her Christmas and her New Year, probably one of the very few she had left. Who can say? What if I had said nothing in spite of the risk and she had sustained a hip fracture?

What if...? She could fracture even with treatment since it takes at least two to three months for the bone to show any healing and even then it is still weak and therefore I could have waited the few days and let her enjoy her holiday. So many difficult questions and so many different answers all of them right...or wrong?

She looked at me, and gave me a weak smile.

"Don't make such a face," she said. "I know you worried about me, but my Christmas was spoiled. I guess such is life!"

I felt like crying.

IS IT DANGEROUS?

Sunday morning, 7:30, the phone rings. I pick up an "urgent" message to call back Mr. Zimmer on the only day of the week I can make up for my chronic lack of sleep. I dial. He picks up after one ring. I picture him in my mind sitting straight up on a chair all dressed up in his three piece suit, looking at the telephone, waiting for it to ring and grabbing it at that first ring. I already know how the conversation will go, as it goes almost every weekend.

"Good morning Mr. Zimmer, what is the problem?" I ask after identifying myself.

"I am sorry to call, but my wife..." he would say in his strongly Hungarian-accented English, "she has had some bad feeling in her stomach since Friday night. Is it dangerous, Doctor?"

"How is she now?"

"Better. Do you think it is the cancer?"

"Tell me first: Did she eat anything this morning?"

"Yes. Less than usual but she ate well enough."

"It does not sound bad. It sounds like whatever she had is going away by itself."

"Then it is not dangerous?"

"No. I don't think so. Keep in touch with me if she has any further problems however."

"Thank you very much doctor. I will tell my wife what you said. It is not dangerous."

"Yes. Good-bye."

That was an exact repetition of many previous similar conversations.

A middle-aged Jewish Hungarian couple, they had come to consult me two years previously because Clara Zimmer had an advanced stage breast cancer. They both had on their forearm the bluish tattoo of a multi-digit number, the telltale sign of their World War II sojourn in a Nazi concentration camp. He had lost his first wife there and she had lost her first husband in a different camp. They had eventually met in the U.S. after the war, got married and had started to build back over the ruins of their lives. Life had then dealt them another blow, breast cancer. Clara had responded very well to treatment but her unfortunate life's experience had conditioned her to say: "Yes, it is well today, but I know it will be bad tomorrow." She was never able to enjoy the months of relief resulting from her treatment.

Because they observed the Sabbath, questions, which arose on Friday, had to be answered before sundown or had to wait till Sunday morning. Mr. Zimmer would not pick up the phone if I called back Friday evening and I could not always call earlier. He was considerate enough however not to call on Saturday night. So, Sunday morning was the time. At first, I was annoyed at being awakened early for a trivial problem on the one day of the week when I occasionally could have a decently long sleep. Clara would never pick up the telephone; her husband was always the one to answer. He was always very polite, concerned and apologetic. I could not be angry with this man in spite of all my internal grumbling. In time I came to the realization that my couple of extra hours of sleep lost were of absolutely no consequence in comparison to the physical and lifelong emotional suffering of these people. On many occasions after this introspective conclusion, I started calling back early on Sunday morning after the Friday call before he felt the need to call me again. Most of the time it was "not dangerous." I even sometimes went back to sleep after making that call and rested even more peacefully for a little while longer because I knew the telephone would not ring and I had taken care of the questions about Clara's problem.

My main regret about the Zimmers has been that I was never able to convince Clara to relax a little and enjoy the time during which she had been free of any symptoms while her cancer had regressed for a period of several months. This experience led me over the years always to emphasize the value of the quality of life for those patients who could enjoy it in spite of their cancer. "Take advantage of the time you feel well," I would always recommend. "When this time is gone, you will have only good memories and no regrets. And if you continue to feel well, enjoy it longer! That is a major reason for the application of any treatment."

Many did indeed follow this advice and were able to experience a worthwhile measure of happiness in spite of their illness.

FORTUNE COOKIE

The love and support of those close to the person who has undergone breast surgery or who is receiving chemotherapy goes a very long way toward healing and tolerating difficult treatment. I don't know whether it prolongs life but it certainly enhances its quality under some very difficult circumstances.

Sharon, a lively young woman who had undergone a mastectomy a few months previously, related to the discussion group she was attending, the event of her arrival home after a few days of hospitalization following the surgery.

"Shortly after I had a chance to get my bearings and to settle again in our home that first night after leaving the hospital, he ravished me as if we were just married. As good as it all was both physically and to my self-image I had to cry for mercy. Sometime later", she added, "I found out that some of the nurses as well as the social worker at the hospital had all talked to him. I gathered later that they had told him that I needed to feel loved more than before because I would feel very self-conscious about my body and my altered conception of my femininity. Well! That is how he interpreted it and that night was quite an experience. We have since settled back into our life. I have no physical hang-ups with him and he does not have to 'ravish' me anymore. The most important thing I want from him is the feeling that he loves me, and I have it."

This young couple had been married for almost ten years. They were obviously very close and occasionally held hands while they talked. She was a petite fiery redhead who used her hands and her whole body when she talked as her face reflected her various emotions. Her husband looked at her with a little smile as she related her experience and her reactions to the surgery and to her illness.

That conversation had taken place years ago at one of the sessions of the support group meeting I had started for patients receiving chemotherapy at a time when the word breast cancer was still uttered only in whispered tones.

"One of the first times I took my wife out for a Chinese dinner after her mastectomy," her husband added as he drew out a slim ribbon of paper from his wallet, "we, of course, opened our fortune cookies at the end of the meal and her fortune said," as he read the little piece of paper he had carried for several months, "*in the eyes of love scars are dimples*. This very simply summarized my feeling about her surgery. Don't think she was not self-conscious about her mastectomy, but she eventually adapted well to the change. So sometime later, at one of our anniversaries, I found a card, that read: '*asymmetry is beautiful*,' and I stuck it on the present I gave her on that occasion. We love one another and nothing will change that."

That, I found over time, is the most valuable component of any treatment for breast cancer.

JOLLY ONCOLOGIST

I had been invited to participate, as member of a panel on breast cancer, in an informative program for a group of women who had been or were presently under treatment for this problem. The session was held at a medical center just outside New York. At six o'clock, members of the audience were finishing the coffee and doughnuts that had been prepared for them and the panelists were gathering at the front row of the small auditorium after having been greeted by our host Dr. Bauer who was to be the moderator of this hour and a half long session. The panel was made up of a breast surgeon, a diagnostic radiologist, a radiation oncologist, a medical oncologist (me) and a plastic surgeon.

The session moved along quite well with the diagnostic radiologist speaking first about the value and techniques of mammography and ultrasound imaging of the breast in the processes of screening for and diagnosis of breast cancer. He spoke about the availability of the various methods of ultrasound guided biopsies of suspicious "shadows" discovered during the course of imaging the breast and how smaller and smaller breast lesions are being discovered at a stage at which cures can be contemplated with appropriate surgical and radiation treatment. He briefly outlined the newer digital and MRI (Magnetic Resonance Imaging) investigative methods of breast cancer detection.

The surgeon spoke about breast self examination, again emphasizing the value of early diagnosis through screening programs. He then went on to explain the options for definitive treatment of the newly discovered breast cancer. He spoke about lumpectomy followed by radiation as well as about mastectomy in situations where it was preferred for special reasons or when lumpectomy was inappropriate. He presented briefly some of the most recent controversies that had arisen in how best to treat the very smallest and earliest of the breast cancers found during the course of screening.

The radiation oncologist spoke about the importance of radiation therapy after lumpectomy for breast cancer explaining that its purpose was the same as the mastectomy, which is to kill any microscopic nests of cancer in that breast instead of removing completely the whole breast potentially containing such tiny clusters of malignant cells. She also talked briefly on the subject of radiation therapy for the treatment of certain metastases, disseminated lesions, that were either very painful or that had the potential for causing serious complications if they progressed any further.

The plastic surgeon explained the fact that mastectomies were still performed often enough and that breast reconstruction could frequently be started at the same time as the mastectomy thus enabling the patient to leave the hospital with a minimum of anatomical disruption. Reconstruction can, of course, be performed at any time after the surgery and he went on to explain the various techniques, which are available, and to show pictures of some of the results of such procedures. One of the two major techniques he described was the one which consists primarily in the implantation of an artificial prosthesis under the chest muscle and by so doing reproducing the shape of a breast on the operated side. A nipple and areola could then be constructed over it in order to complete the appearance of a breast. The other technique was the one which consists in using the patient's own tissue from another part of the body to reconstruct a breast. He spoke about the possible problems associated with each but explained that the majority of these procedures went without any complications. There were a lot of questions from the audience this being a major concern of women who had undergone mastectomy, a good proportion of whom had not elected or were still hesitant about undergoing an additional surgical procedure.

My turn to speak was the last and the more arduous because the topic I was to cover concerned not only the treatment of women with a good prognosis, those who were already potentially cured of their cancer by surgery but also and particularly those whom I treated because they had passed the curable stage of their breast cancer by virtue of the fact that their disease had disseminated itself in their body.

I emphasized both the curability of those who having completed their surgery received (adjuvant) chemotherapy in order to decrease the risk of appearance of disseminated lesions, and the tractability of those whose cancer was no longer curable. I dwelt particularly on the effectiveness of the many available forms of treatment of metastatic breast cancer as well as on the existing methods of preventing and minimizing many of the most uncomfortable side effects of the chemotherapy. I illustrated the last point by describing our so-called "rogues gallery" of Polaroid pictures of our patients eating their sandwiches and drinking their coffee while the intravenous bags of toxic chemotherapeutic medications with noxious-sounding names were dripping into their veins. I spoke about our total intolerance to side effects whereby we the physicians stated jokingly that we would get "conniption fits" if they happened and that our patients were therefore requested to be kind enough to try very hard to spare us that experience. I also told them that we would arrange to have their hair grow back red and curly after the chemotherapy and how we were planning to patent that process for those who wanted such hair, and similar nonsense we would go through in order to lighten up the process of chemotherapy.

I related how the seriousness of the chemotherapy sessions can be relaxed such as on the occasion of my son's birthday. He was also my associate in our oncology practice. On that day one of our patients came for her chemotherapy session bringing him a beautiful birthday ice cream cake. She insisted that he cut it right there and then. So, he proceeded to do it only to find that, hard as he tried, the knife would not go through its icing. He thought it was frozen solid. After a few minutes of futile effort, he finally discovered that it was made of a roll of paper towel dipped in plaster, dried, colored and shaped like an elaborate cake covered with icing and candles. Everyone had a good laugh and the chemotherapy session went on.

These little mirth-producing ploys don't always work. I related a time when having returned from an international breast cancer meeting in China I came up with another idea to make my patients smile. Hot flashes are a common complaint during treatment, be it hormonal or chemotherapeutic. Estrogens, the most specific treatment of this symptom are still avoided because of their potential for stimulating breast cancer. So when one of my regular patients complained again about that symptom at her follow up visit on that day I explained to her that I had brought back from my trip some wonderful Chinese folk medicine for it. It always worked, I added, and had no undesirable side effects, no dose limitation and I then proceeded to offer her one of these small Chinese folding paper fans, hand painted with a colorful bird on one side and a flower on the other. I had a box full of them. She burst out laughing. Over the next few days I repeated the same innocuous joke for a couple of other women with the same reaction. One of them however looked at me unsmiling and said: "We are not amused!" In retrospect this had to be expected in her case. She was very unhappy in her personal life. Menopausal symptoms increased her unhappiness and no attempt at a light joke was going to help this. I recognized my mistake, and my apology was formally accepted.

While I told the audience about ongoing funny exchanges which went on between the patients and our staff, I talked mainly about the significant and hopefully increasing number of long-term survivors with good quality of life, among those women treated for a disseminated disease generally felt to be incurable. I dwelt heavily on the fact that while effective methods of treatment were available and their side effects were manageable, treatment of cancer in general and of breast cancer in particular is a constantly evolving field with new, different and, many times, potentially more effective forms of treatment, appearing at increasingly shorter intervals.

At the end of this meeting I gathered my slides and walked to the elevator where I found a woman who had attended this meeting already waiting for it.

"You are a rather jolly oncologist," she said as I arrived.

"Why not?" I replied. "Life is not easy for those receiving chemotherapy for cancer and neither is it simple for those of us who administer it. If together we can mix some humor with the treatment it makes it both more acceptable and more tolerable at the receiving end and less stressful at the delivery side."

"I also receive chemotherapy, but at the hospital," she informed me. "My oncologist, who is very good and whom I respect deeply, is so serious and so gloomy all the time that he depresses me. He tells me, or I gather from what he says, that the treatment I receive will not make any difference in the long run. How can you laugh or joke with all this?"

"I can because people can, because I am truly optimistic, because I emphasize the success of our treatment efforts in spite of their limitations, because I know that success can happen often enough even if it is not all the time. That is why I do what I do the way I do it. Optimism is a major ingredient in the practice of oncology. Humor also helps."

"Well I must say this is certainly a different way of looking at things and I feel I can have a different outlook on the treatment I am receiving in spite of my depressive physician. I truly enjoyed your presentation."

"And you gave me an idea," I replied. "If I can find someone to design it I will fly the Jolly Oncologist flag over our door."

We both laughed as we parted.

THE SMILE

May Sullivan looked suddenly worried as I finished examining her and telling her she could now get dressed.

She did not move from the examining table.

"What is wrong with me doctor?" she asked. "Did you find anything bad?"

She seemed frightened.

"No. What makes you think that?" I truly had found her well. This had been a routine follow up examination months after she had completed her course of chemotherapy. She remained quite healthy. All her blood tests had been normal and the most recent imaging studies, x-rays and scans had all revealed nothing remotely worrisome.

"You did not smile," she said. "You always smile when you see me. I got worried."

"Oh for heavens sake! Was that it?" Now, I truly had to smile. "I had some problems on my mind today, totally unrelated to you. That took my smile away temporarily early in the day. I guess it had not yet managed to return. You, however, are fine. I am sorry I worried you."

"I don't know how you do it, Doctor. How can you go on all day like this and smile most of the time and put up with people like me? How do you do it? Don't you get depressed?"

"No, I don't. I do it because the rewards are great. There is no greater feeling than to see someone who was seriously ill a few weeks ago come back truly improved as result of my treatment. Not that treatment is always successful but the victories amply compensate for the times of heartaches and failures. That is why I do what I do and why I can smile."

On that occasion, I truly realized the impact of body language on the people I cared for. A smile, a frown, a gesture, a look, a single word in a sentence, are all things they read and interpret in their own way. I, in turn, have to look for their reaction to my attitude lest something I did or said be interpreted the wrong way as it had been on that day.

MY TURN, MY BOOST

The tables turned one morning when Madeline K. greeted me and asked me how I felt. I gave the standard answer: "I feel quite well, thank you. No use complaining, no one listens anyway," I added.

"Not so," she said. "I listen and I am concerned about you. You are the one always asking how we are doing, what problems we have, how we do with the treatment. I know you worry and you work very hard and so I also worry about you. You take good care of me and I want you to also take care of yourself, not only because I like you but also because I need you to be well. Take some time off and rest."

I was truly taken by surprise. No one ever asks me how I am, truly, how I really feel. Not that I miss it but it was nice to find someone who seemed to care for me, care enough to ask not simply as a greeting but as a question arising from concern even though the motive was acknowledged to be also in part selfish.

My mood was uplifted and I felt very well the rest of that day.

ROSES

I did not know her. She had come for her regular annual checkup by my old friend and surgical colleague who shared our office for a few months. She carried a magnificent bouquet of two dozens of the most beautiful long stem red roses I had seen, accompanied by a large smile. She presented both to him and gave him a hug.

"What was the occasion?" I asked his secretary after she had left.

"It is a story that started twenty-four years ago," she told me. "When Connie consulted Dr. A. for the first time she had a large mass in her right breast. She had watched it grow for a few months and had finally decided to do something about it. You know my boss. He was about to give her hell for waiting so long to show up but the poor soul was so scared he gave her only purgatory and scheduled her for a radical mastectomy and postoperative radiation therapy."

That was still the standard initial treatment at the time.

The secretary continued: "She was so scared to die and so thankful for his care that she did not know what she could do to thank him. She was so grateful she wanted to give him a beautiful present but did not know what he liked. When she finally asked him after a few visits to his office he told her he only wanted her to bring him roses once a year and each time the number of roses should amount to the number of years she had been alive and doing well. That day was the twenty fourth anniversary of her surgery."

SECTION V
BEYOND THE WALL

****

It was easier for the physician at a time, years ago, when all he had to say was "Do as I say, everything will be fine" or "it just has to get a little worse before it gets better," and other such things that patients expected to hear and never questioned. It was an easy way out of a heart-breaking conversation about how things really were. In some countries, the omnipotence of the physician persists to this day, including parts of the industrialized western world. In the United States, this attitude started changing in the late fifties and sixties and it has taken it several years to reach the point at which the word cancer may be used in conversation, treatment and prognosis can be discussed openly and even the ultimate end of this potentially fatal illness can be discussed, albeit very carefully, every word and sentence being considered with forethought before being actually spoken. Such a conversation is still and naturally associated with a very strong emotional component affecting both the patient and the physician.

An easy way out for the physician who does not wish to be subjected to the strain of discussing terminal treatment and death is to hide behind statistical figures such as: "Twenty percent will respond, eighty percent will not. What else can I tell you?"

Or, "there is nothing else I can offer you but I can refer you for hospice care, they will handle all that is needed."

That does not answer the questions of: "How bad this is going to be? Am I going to be in more pain? Am I dying? Isn't there anything else? What happens when I die? How does it happen? What do I do if my mother dies at home? Who do I call? What about if it happens at night? Do I call you? Should she be hospitalized?"

It is certainly easier to have someone else at the receiving end of these questions because the physician who gives the opportunity to the patient and her family to ask these questions must have gone through the exercise of asking these same questions of himself or herself and must have thought long and frequently about the answers. He or she must have addressed mentally, and logically, his or her own vulnerability to serious illness and his or her own mortality. It is only then that such a physician becomes able to listen to all these questions, talk openly about them and formulate answers that can be adapted to the multiplicity of clinical and psychosocial settings presented by the patient.

What happens when the cancer and its treatment have reached the impenetrable wall which marks the limits of our ability to treat? A wall so high that one can only guess what is beyond it and yet one that, for all its apparent forbidding strength, is the one that has been periodically moved further and further away during cancer treatment. What happens when it is reached? Does one try to scale it through investigational therapies? Does on just lie at its base, bare to the elements, awaiting death? Does one seek help to build a shelter such as to avail oneself of whatever comfort until such time as death comes as the ultimate relief? What about the traveler's companions, those she or he has cared for all along and who may be left alone through the rest of life's journey?

How long before it is reached does one anticipate the presence of this wall? How far ahead does one look for the location of this ultimate structure? How strongly does one hope that by the time its anticipated location is reached it might have been moved further away? All the questions that the physician has already been asked many times and waits for the next patient to ask, and when appropriate sometimes discretely encouraging the initiation of such a discussion.

In this time of high-tech, "virtual reality" concepts, this wall is both virtual and real. We shall all face it sooner or later. For many people who have experienced the impact of cancer at a fortunately early stage in its development to be curable, the concept is more virtual. For those in whom this disease reaches the non curable stage it is closer to being real although it does not truly become concrete until later.

This section relates events and conversations resulting from the set of circumstances in which the "wall," or the mythological River Styx, no longer limited to a concept, becomes visible in the distance.

HOPE

———

"What next? Is there anymore treatment for me?"

"There is always something that can be done" has always been my usual answer.

"But you have already given me four different types of treatment, hormones and chemotherapy, you tell me that my cancer has worsened again and I have more pain. What now?"

Catherine Mullen had walked in to my consultation with a slight limp and in a way she was right. I was fast exhausting the therapeutic possibilities available for the management of her metastatic breast cancer. There were still one or two treatment options left that offered a possibility, though small, of producing further temporary arrest or regression of the cancer. She might also be included in one or the other of a limited number of investigational programs. I had tried to get her into one of them previously but the program had already closed having obtained the number of patients required for the data to be statistically valid. In another trial they wanted only patients who had previously received no more than one course of chemotherapy and consequently she did not qualify for it.

"First of all I have already planned the next form of chemotherapy for you and I will tell you the details of it later. The drug I propose to use already has a track record of effectiveness in people who have failed the chemotherapies you have already received. We have used it in our practice with some good results bearing in mind that it does not always work but it is quite well tolerated and therefore worth a try."

"What are the percentages?"

"You mean what is the likelihood that this treatment will work. In general, reports indicate that about thirty percent of all those treated are expected to respond. This percentage is smaller those who have already received a lot of chemotherapy and may vary according to the number of different treatment regimens received. Basically, however, it will either work or it will not, whatever the percentages. What I have to emphasize is that the reason for treating is to produce a regression of the cause of your discomfort. That is the most effective mechanism of relief. If it works, in the balance you will feel definitely better."

"What if it does not?" she pursued.

"Then, unfortunately, you will have received the treatment for naught again bearing in mind that without treatment the cancer and its associated discomfort is sure to increase. With treatment there is still a real possibility of improvement."

She thought for a moment, and then asked, "What about simply taking pain medications? That can give good relief without all the discomfort of the chemotherapy."

"Indeed, it can. Still, if it stops the growth of the cancer, specific anticancer treatment gives the best form of symptom relief for as long as it works. Pain medications may have to be used until it starts working. But yes, there will be... there is a time when pain medications and other forms of symptom relief become the best and only course to follow when anticancer medications have little more to offer.

"So, when all treatments fail and you have nothing more to treat me with, pain medications can still be of help?"

"They certainly can. At that time, truly, symptom control becomes the main course to follow and that can be achieved effectively by several means. My concern is primarily you, you who harbor that cancer. You are the one who guides me in accepting my recommendations regarding one course of action or another, one set of medications or another."

"I am glad you are explaining this to me but still I know that the choices for treatment are very few at this time."

"You are right at this time but let me point out some facts to you. The treatment of breast cancer, or of any cancer for that matter has not been cast in stone ten years ago never to change. It is constantly changing. Every few months information comes out about new drugs, new ways of using already existing drugs, different sequences of treatments as well as totally new concepts in treatment. As a matter of fact the medication

I propose to start you on next was not available until only fairly recently and other new methods are already visible in the very foreseeable future. The entire strategy is designed to gain time until something else comes around and, like in a chess game, to plan several steps ahead and also be ready to change this plan based on changing circumstances. With all this I understand your question and your concern. Your concern is that at our present state of knowledge there will come a time when there will not be any worthwhile treatment available. Or what will be available will have such a low probability of being effective and such a high probability of causing severe side effects that its usefulness in helping you will be very questionable. What then? At that time treatment will continue but along a different line. While until then it will have been directed specifically against the cancer itself, at that time it will become directed toward the control of the cancer symptoms: relief of pain and of anxiety, maintenance of nutrition, digestion, elimination, comfort in breathing, in short maintenance of *general comfort*. That is part and parcel of the treatment of cancer and it is good treatment by itself at the appropriate time as well as during the course of any chemotherapy."

"Thank you for explaining all this to me. I read and hear all about the horrors of dying with cancer, I remember the suffering my aunt went through before she died and I can tell you now that I have lived in terror of this. Can you really keep me remain comfortable at the end? That is truly all I want to be sure of."

Catherine is a religious woman. She goes to church and I am sure that, among other things, she prays to be spared the severe suffering she fears so much. Physical distress is dreaded and yet it is taught and seen by some as both the path to redemption and eternal bliss and also as the ultimate punishment for the evil deed of the sinners. The practice of self-induced suffering from simply giving up certain gratifications to the extreme of self flagellation becomes for some a form of bargain with their Creator, inducing predictable suffering in their lifetime as advanced payment for the privilege and quasi assurance of eternal bliss and rest in the hereafter. And so, Catherine prays to be spared and has faith that God will look after her. She also has faith in her physician's ability to spare her the agony she fears. And all I can do is try and hope that whatever treatment I apply will do just that. All I can do is watch week after week for signs of regression of the cancer, coax her and encourage her to put up with her symptoms and with the problems of the treatment until the glorious day when the most recent examination and tests confirm another victory in the long war against her cancer or until the day when, like a toll, the findings indicate a failure of the therapy and signal the need to reassess the diminishing therapeutic options.

"I can assure you that I can and I will," I answered, "but you are not at the end yet and, if you let me, I plan to try very hard to make you better. I wish you also to remember a thing you must be already aware of: No treatment is imposed upon you. You play a most important role in planning the strategy of your care and that is why I take the time to explain to you why I make certain recommendations and consider certain other alternatives. This way you can tell me whether to go ahead or to do something else with full understanding of the benefits, the limitations and the problems you will be facing. It is always your choice to start, to continue or to stop any treatment. My job is to make selections, make the recommendations and explain them to you, it is to steer you along an optimal course through the storms of your illness and find shelters from them. Throughout this voyage we shall both accentuate the positive and plan for a good outcome. I plan to go on with you to the finishing line all the while trying together to push it back."

"When you talk to me you always make me feel better, more hopeful and more positive. I will make the appointments to start the chemotherapy whenever you say."

There is always hope and yet hope takes many forms with different goals at different times and at different stages of the disease. There is the hope that the breast lump just found is not cancerous. If it is found to be cancerous the hope is that it may be curable when treated. If it is not cured and spreads in the body the hope is that it can be treated successfully and made to regress, hopefully for a very long time. When it relapses again the hope is that something better or new may help again and if that fails over and over the hope is that suffering can be relieved and controlled. When pain and anguish last too long the final hope is that death will come as a relief without more suffering. The final hope is that the mystery of the hereafter is truly the entrance to eternal peace.

For some, structured religion is a great source of comfort, hope, and peace. For others, it can be cause for more anxiety. Those for whom a philosophy defining life as part of the universe has replaced an organized and structured religion, meditation can bring the same degree of hope and peace. There is invariably a time when even the most skeptics among us go through a metaphysical resurgence of the mind when the end of life is approaching. This spiritual resurgence is very important in the process of living through the transit from life to death. It frequently crystallizes one's thoughts about the purpose of the rest of that life and one's appreciation of all its components. It promotes a peaceful emotional state when the end of the journey is reached. The physician's help in this process, conveyed through open communication, is invaluable.

I AM TOO YOUNG

Miriam's breast cancer journey had been stormy from the start and it was close to ending with no safe harbor in sight. She was 29 and had been fighting it for the previous two years. She was a single, bright, working young woman. The cancer was an aggressive one from the very start. The lump had appeared and grown over a period of a few weeks. Metastases appeared soon after she had completed her course of adjuvant chemotherapy and her response to additional treatment on three more occasions had been disappointing. Responses had been very short with each new medication and the last attempt at chemotherapy had been a complete failure. She has recently enrolled in a trial of immunotherapy with a breast cancer vaccine that was being tested in order to find the dose that could be administered safely, to study its side effects and to determine whether any benefits could be observed, as they had been in experimental animals. She was ready for it. She was to receive it at the cancer center but she came to see me periodically for comfort and direction in case it failed.

"Look at me," she said with tears running down her cheeks, "here I am only 29 years old and, while my girl friends talk about going out, having fun, dating, getting married or expecting a baby, I think I am going to die soon. Why is that?"

I had no good answer. I just held her hand and agreed that life had been very unfair.

The treatment trial went on and she continued to see me periodically. She was responding. The cancer was regressing. She started feeling better although she often developed fever for a couple of days after each injection of the vaccine.

While that went on she met a young man with whom she became quite close. He accompanied her at her visits to my office every few weeks. One day, she announced that they were planning to get married within a couple of months.

"He asked me and I said yes," she told me when she announced the news. "I have little time and I want to have some of the taste of a normal life while I still can. It will be very little but I want to have experienced it before I die."

Shortly thereafter, her condition stopped improving and she started getting weaker. But the marriage took place as planned one evening at her home. It was small event attended mostly by members of her family and one or two close friends. My wife and I were also invited.

All eyes were moist when she appeared in her white dress with flowers in her wig and stood beside her groom as the religious ceremony proceeded and as he crushed the glass under his foot according to the Jewish tradition, and as wishes for long life and happiness were expressed.

Miriam died within three months of her wedding

Her legacy to others was that the last treatment gave one of the first proofs that there was an entirely new and promising approach to the treatment of breast cancer. Shad responded to the vaccine treatment and that response, short as it had been, had given the medical world a glimpse of new treatments to come.

Miriam's story confirmed in my mind the idea that breast cancer is not a single disease but is composed of a group of cancers that produce an entire spectrum of clinical courses. At one end of that spectrum one cancer can be very slow growing and regresses with almost any treatment, while at the other is another cancer that responds to none and that moves on inexorably. All of them are called breast cancer. One of these days, it will become possible to identify* these different clinical behaviors at the onset of the disease and target the treatment to each particular tumor based on that information.

Nowadays this is indeed taking place as a result of the genetic identifications and several other biological characters of breast cancer(s).

MY WILL BE DONE?

Blair was a wealthy, divorced, business woman who had first consulted me when her breast cancer was already far advanced and she had been referred to me in search of a last resort treatment in the hope of getting some relief of her pains and hope of healing of the metastases that had progressed to the state of open sores on her chest.

The chemotherapy had worked again and she had begun to feel better. She was particularly happy about the progress of the healing of the open sores. She was now planning to return to Florida where she resided and where she was the CEO of a profitable business.

She came one day to my office accompanied by her sister who was at the time a prominent personality in the national political circles. When they finally sat down in my office after her treatment I explained to her sister Blair's condition and discussed the anticipated course of the cancer. When I was done with my cautiously realistic description of a progressive breast cancer Blair broke in with her questions.

"I understand this cancer will eventually get me," she said, "but because of it, I have some concerns of a different nature. How much time do you think I have?"

People had frequently asked me that question as a way to ask me if I expected them to die soon without addressing the question of death directly. I have usually responded by asking a question of my own as I did again on that occasion. "Why do you want to know?" I asked her in turn. "Do you just want to know out of curiosity or does your question have a specific purpose?"

"Yes, there is a specific reason for my question. I want to revise my will and wish to know whether I have enough time to do that."

When confronted with that question I usually try to redirect and clarify the question by asking if that is indeed a way of asking me how long I think tat person has to live, for if that is its purpose I cannot give a time limit. On the other hand, if the question is generated by a genuine concern about putting affairs in order, my answer remains always the same.

And that is how I continued with Blair: "No one can tell you how long you have to live. However, if you are concerned about your present will not reflecting your present wishes in its existing structure or, if you have not yet prepared any will and you are concerned about how your inheritance will be disposed of, then by all means get it done and put you mind at ease. Then, if you die soon, it will have been taken care of and you will not have to worry until that happens. If you live for a long time you may want to change it again sometime along the way but until then your mind will be at ease, at least as far as that is concerned. Don't do it because your think you will soon be dead, do it because it is a task that is pending and that you want to complete."

"OK, well put," she said. "But now I have another question. As you know, I am the CEO of the company my father started and I have been running it for many years after he died. I work with very dependable people but I have to think about whether to continue in my present position or should I plan to resign and pass the direction of this company to someone else?"

"That," I answered, "is something you must decide by yourself. Do you think that at this moment you feel well enough to continue to carry the work you have been doing at your company and, if you are, for now, do you think this will continue?"

She thought for only a brief moment.

"You are right," she said. "I have felt this way for a while but kept talking myself out of it." She looked at her sister. "Don't you think he is right?" she asked. Her sister nodded in acquiescence as she dried her eyes with her small handkerchief.

Most people know the answer to the type of questions put before me by Blair that day. They seek both reassurance and confirmation. The unknown is often more frightening than the reality. Confirmation and explanation, of even the worse scenario, afford a degree of peace of mind because the question is finally answered, the mystery is unveiled, often revealing that the fantasy that is built about it is often worse than the reality. One can then move on to the business of dealing with it, of adjusting to its revealed inevitability and no longer guessing and fearing it. At that time, it becomes possible to seek the reassurance needed to sustain one through the difficult and dangerous path ahead, mostly the reassurance that no matter what lies ahead, help, support, and relief will be at hand until the end.

IS IT WORTH IT?

Isabel was wheeled into our office for her first consultation and, by all criteria, she fitted the category of patients about whom many colleagues would say, "What's the use," meaning that nothing useful will be accomplished with treatment at that stage of the illness.

I was upset at the fact that I had not been forewarned of her precarious condition for, had I known it, I would have planned to hospitalize her directly without putting her through the discomfort of coming first to my office and then have to be transferred, if by luck there was a bed available at the hospital, or to have to return home and then prepare for her admission at a later date.

She could not walk without pain because of the extent of the spread of the cancer in her bones. She could not see straight for the previous two to three days because metastases inside her head had compressed one of the nerves that controls the movements of one of her eyes and, by the time I received her laboratory reports later that day, it was clear that her breast cancer had reach the stage of its progression at which it interfered with her calcium metabolism, causing it to rise to a toxic level in her blood.

Sensing the desperate state of her condition she refused to be hospitalized for the urgently needed treatment, preferring to remain at home with her two small children and her husband to the end. She said that she would accept any recommended treatment and that she would go for any necessary tests as long as these could be done without hospitalization.

Treatment was started on the day she first came with a combination of chemotherapy and a hormonal medication in addition to which analgesics were prescribed in order to relieve her pain.

The plan was to follow her closely at first, at weekly intervals. We kept in touch by telephone on a daily basis. At her next visit a week later she volunteered the information that her pain was greatly improved and when her eyes were tested it was obvious that movements of her affected eye were almost back to normal. Within a month she was walking with the support of a walker. Four months later she had returned to work in her office job and her husband who had taken time off to care for her was able to return to his teaching job.

"When I first came," she told one day, "I could not even think straight and all I could think was if all that effort was really worth it; and here I am back to work. But what is really worth all of it is that I can take care of my two kids and be with them. That is worth anything."

It lasted two and a half years and then one day, when she came for her follow up visit I could clearly see that things had changed. She looked suddenly tired and had lost weight within a few weeks. When I examined her, I found that her liver had enlarged and I could feel the tumor lumps that had grown in it. From then on no treatment could stop it. No response was obtained with any of the anticancer medications I administered to her over the next several weeks.

A few months after she had died her parents and her husband came to see me and to tell me how important had been the couple of years she had been able to return to an almost normal life. It had been particularly important to her children who were able to grow a little longer with the presence of their mother. And while her parents mourned their child and her husband his wife, they were all grateful for the little additional time they had been able be together. It had all been truly worth it.

I always wore on my lapel the little angel pin they gave me in her memory.

Throughout my career as an oncologist, colleagues, friends and patients' relatives have asked me how I could go on day after day treating so many people whose illness is frequently incurable. My answer has been that I work with a different set of goals. If a cure cannot be achieved, prolongation of purposeful life, maintaining the quality of that life, in comfort, with the element of hope * always in the background, are all worthwhile goals. Limited victories such as that achieved for Isabel amply make up for the frequent ultimate defeats.

* Read chapter: HOPE.

LET ME DIE

I went to see Tara at her home on that snowy February night after completing my office hours and my hospital rounds. She had become too weak to travel to my office and a hospice care program had been organized for her at home. I had not seen her in four weeks and I had decided to make a detour by Brooklyn before getting home that evening.

Only a bedside lamp lit the bedroom. Tara was in her bed in semi-seated position amidst a number of cushions and pillows of various sizes, shapes and colors. Her husband was seated beside her and was holding her hand. She looked gaunt, thinner than her usual already thin body-build. Her face was deeply furrowed. She looked at me very intensely.

"Let me die already," she said. "It's enough! I cannot live like this! I don't want to live like this! Make it end already."

A request I understood and could not ignore in the face of the fact that she had already undergone all the therapeutic procedures usually applied to the treatment of metastatic breast cancer as well as some of the newest chemotherapies specifically used in that clinical complex. She was neither a candidate for, nor did she wish to participate in any investigational treatment program. She was exhausted. She had had it! I had treated her for her advanced cancer for over ten years. Treatment had made it regress initially for almost seven years. She had enjoyed these, had worked through them, and had danced through them, dance having been her favorite and most important pass-time. Then when it flared up again it was brought back under control for several months. Each time it flared up again it responded but for decreasing periods. Now it was no longer responding to any anti-cancer medications. Radiation therapy and treatment with a radioactive isotope had controlled some of the local bone pains for a while but now it was no longer possible to move her to apply any more radiation and pain was progressive. Her liver was almost totally replaced by tumor.

"Tell me why you want to end it all now?" I asked.

"Because I am in pain and it is not getting better and besides, what else can you do for me?"

"If I can make you free or almost free of pain would you be satisfied?"

"Yes, but I still want out. I don't want this life anymore. I stay in the room, I don't see anyone, I cannot walk, I cannot dance, I cannot move in bed, this is not living. I might as well be dead. I want to die!"

"I understand, but hear me out. I cannot make you die but I can make you pain-free for whatever period of life you have left. Is that an acceptable compromise for you?"

"All right, I have no choice. Tell me how to do it."

"I understand from your husband that you take your pain medication only if the pain becomes unbearable. That is the wrong way to take it."

"It makes me groggy," she protested. "If I take more I cannot think."

"I know but if you take it on a regular around-the-clock schedule the grogginess will eventually subside and you will maintain the pain control. And if you are still a little bit groggy so be it! It is still better than being in pain all the time. Don't you think so?" I argued.

"I guess so."

"I will increase the strength of the long acting pain patch that you put on every seventy two hours. Continue to take the pills every four hours for the next two to three days. It will take that long to increase the level of these medications in your blood stream. If you find that you have experienced good pain relief after the two to three days, decrease the frequency of the pills to every five to six hours. It is possible that after a while the larger dose of medication in the skin patch will be sufficient by itself to keep you quite comfortable. If that does not work well enough, the dose may be increased further until it is satisfactory. Call me every two to three days to tell me how it goes and I will tell you what adjustments to make."

"OK, but I still want to die," she insisted.

"I know but, short of death, comfort is not a bad thing to achieve and *that* I can do for you. There is something else I want you to do and that is to open your curtains and your windows a little during the day to let in light and fresh air. At night, I want you to have some bright lighting in you bedroom until you are ready to go to sleep. If your pain gets relieved enough with the right doses of the pain medications, I want you to ask your daytime helper to assist you in sitting on the wheelchair and push you in front of the window in order to enable you to look at the outside world."

"I will try all that but tell me please, how will I die? Will I suffer?"

"Not if I can help it and if you follow my instructions. What will happen is that over a period of time you will start feeling increasingly tired and sleepy. Eventually you will sleep most of the time and the next step will be all the time. When this happens dying will be a very small step away and you will be feeling nothing uncomfortable. No one has come back to tell if there is more to it but my best perception of this process is that suffering is not part of it. As a matter of fact you may well start feeling better soon."

That was what would be expected with the relentless failure of her liver function. What I did not add is that, not infrequently, the dying person will suddenly feel totally comfortable shortly before death. On several occasions, patients have described to me a feeling of total peace and euphoria for a few hours or a day before they died. In many of these instances they have called their relatives to say good-bye and when all was done they closed their eyes in a restful eternal sleep.

I sat at Tara's side for a few minutes. I finally got up.

"I will go now," I said. "But I will keep in touch with you, your husband or your nurse daily."

I found very early in my medical career that I could talk to my patients about death without being self-conscious and without feeling the need to deny its evident imminence. The patients in turn have felt comfortable talking to me about their concerns and fears about the transit to the end of their life. When they question me about it some look for words reassuring them that this end is not imminent but all of them look for information about this final step from life into the unknown that is death. Most of them know when the time for their ultimate passage is close. That is mostly when they ask for the assurance that this final process of their life will proceed without any terrible suffering.

The room was suddenly silent as Tara processed my recommendations in her mind. Her husband was still seated at her side holding her hand.

"All right," she finally exclaimed, "but may I call you if I have a problem?"

"Of course you can. As I already told you, I want to hear from you daily in order to make sure you don't need anything else."

Tara took her medications as prescribed. She did not get into the wheelchair but whenever the weather was not too cold, her windows were opened to let in a bit of fresh air during the day. Her pain improved markedly and was almost totally relieved over the next few days. She slowly lapsed into a coma due to the rapid deterioration of her liver by the tumor metastases and died peacefully shortly thereafter. She just stopped breathing.

She had been a musician and a ballroom dancer. As long as she was well she danced two to three times a week. When she could no longer dance because any exertion exacerbated the pain of her bone metastases she considered her life to be over and for her it was although it was not the pain itself that brought her to that point, it was the loss of independence, the end of joy, the limitation of purpose that did it.

WAS IT A DREAM?

Tell me Doctor, could I die of this?"

I have had to answer this question probably no more than a total of half a dozen times during my professional life. I mean this question with "I" as the subject, not "could my wife" or "could my sister die soon." This question was asked by the patient herself on these rare occasions when it had become obvious to her that her condition had truly become desperate, that all previous treatments had failed and that there were truly no worthwhile therapeutic options left. This question, when asked, came as her acknowledgement that her life was close to its end. Yes, one could always try something else, but it was acknowledged by both of us that such a trial would be a futile gesture more likely to disrupt than to improve the quality of the balance of her life.

What could I say in the face of what we both knew was obvious, while preserving at the same time the emotional integrity of that person?

"Yes," I answered each time. "That could happen".

"Soon?"

"Yes, it could be soon".

"How soon?" was her next and most difficult question.

"Oh, I truly cannot tell. Is it important for you to know the time?"

"Not really. I thought you could tell."

"It could be days, weeks or even some months".

"Many months?"

"Probably not but one may be very surprised sometimes. The cancer may remain stable for a while and so, any time limit that I could state is a guess."

"But it may be very soon. Yes?"

"Yes. It may be".

She was silent for a while and we sat there side by side rather than on both sides of the barrier of my desk between us.

"Tell me," she then said, "You have seen people die. What is it like?"

I have often thought about death but never in a morbid way.

Even as an adolescent or a young man, I never contemplated death as a frightening experience. In time, I explored books on the subject of the change from life to death and long ago viewed it as part of the continuum of existence. I did not and do not view death as the end of anything but as a natural sequence to life as commonly defined and more as a unidirectional unstoppable sequence of transitions through time and the universe of which we are all an integral part.

What I could tell this middle aged woman who was preparing for the ultimate transition was only a perception I had one afternoon in my early twenties, a perception, that to this day, remains in my memory as a feeling of floating somewhere between dream and reality. As I napped one summer afternoon I suddenly turned around, in my dream I thought later, and saw myself lying on the couch in my room. I saw myself very clearly for a very brief instant after which all turned black and empty. I was surrounded by blackness dotted with millions of tiny bright lights. There was no sound, no sensation of my body, nothing except for an utter feeling of peace and rest I had never experienced before or since. Was it a dream? Did I die for a very short instant? I will never know but this memory has remained with me as my concept of the moment of death.

Without describing the circumstances of this experience, I have, on the few occasions when the question was placed before me, tried to pass on the feeling I had on that day as a likely one of the moment of death. Those I have talked to about it appeared relieved and appeased and for myself I feel at peace with that feeling.

EPILOGUE

THE CRYSTAL BALL AND THE TIME MACHINE

****

Many times, one or the other of those patients under my care asks me if any progress has been achieved in the fight against breast cancer and what the future may bring. Every so often, the news media relate the fact that with all the so-called progress women still die of breast cancer, that progress is slow to change that, that it is still a prevalent disease, that its cause is still obscure, that there are not enough funds devoted to research in that field... so what has happened, what is truly happening, and what will happen?

My answers to this are directed to what has happened in the past and what is already foreseeable for the future. Traveling in the past through the time machine of my aging brain I recall the time when for a woman breast cancer meant having to undergo a radical mastectomy almost always followed by radiation therapy to the mastectomy area of the chest wall and the armpit. Cancer was still an illness one did not mention by name and breast cancer was the perceived end of femininity for the person involved. Surgeons have been blamed for their surgical savaging of women's bodies at a time when, by applying the state of the art treatment of their time as best they knew, many women have been completely and permanently *cured* of that cancer. The complications of the treatment were common and represented the aftermath of the combination of the radical surgery and the radiation.

But major progress has occurred. Several years ago, as a result of a large study on the usefulness of screening mammography, earlier and smaller breast cancers began to be discovered. Later, thanks to two "political" breast cancers that afflicted two very courageous women, Happy Rockefeller and Betty Ford, that illness was brought out of the closet. These two women were in the political limelight and by publicizing their personal experiences they encouraged other women to take action instead of hiding their breast lumps until it was too late for a cure to be achieved. Women started to ask for mammography and physicians themselves had to become educated in that respect. That took time, but it happened. This led to trials of less extensive surgery for the earlier, smaller cancers and now most breast cancers are treated with breast conservation while mastectomy is performed increasingly rarely. Over the same period of time, the developments in the technology of radiation therapy viewed through the same time machine have been such that better results with minimal complications due to the radiation itself have been achieved. The telltale, swollen arm that was a frequent complication of the traditional radical mastectomy is now rarely seen with the more conservative surgery.

More importantly, the diagnosis of very small cancers made possible by screening mammography has increased the cure rate of breast cancer and has opened the way to less extensive surgical procedures. With the help of new imaging technology and imaginative physicians, explorations of even more limited procedures are under way to replace, in selected clinical situations the primary surgical ablation of the initial breast tumor. Such investigative techniques involve imaging-guided probes which may destroy very small tumors by heat, freezing or high frequency energy devices.

Furthermore, based upon technological progress and upon a better understanding of this cancer's biology the primary treatment of breast cancer is no longer limited to the local procedure consisting of surgery with or without radiation. While in the past, one waited for the traditional other shoe to fall, meaning for metastases to appear before starting any systemic treatment for breast cancer, nowadays a systemic treatment is frequently part of this primary treatment and it is administered in the form of either hormonal and/or cytotoxic chemotherapy. Such treatment is based on the likelihood that, given certain morphological and biological characteristics, a breast cancer may have a greater or lesser chance of having already spread microscopically by the time it is found in the breast. This, in turn, has contributed to change the spectrum of the disease.

As a result of all the above cures are more likely to occur after the local treatment of the primary breast tumor. The interval between the diagnosis of the malignancy and the first clinical evidence of spread of the disease to sites distant from the breast, known as the disease-free interval, has been prolonged. Overall survival has been prolonged. Some types of metastases such as the diffusely ulcerated chest wall lesions, that were frequent in the past, are now seen very rarely. A previously frequent metabolic complication of breast cancer, an elevation of the serum calcium to toxic levels in the blood, has also become rare. It is possible that the early application of a generalized form of treatment may have eliminated from the breast cancer cell population those clones that caused these particular complications.

New forms of hormonal treatment, administered orally and/or by injection, have replaced the previous surgical methods that were designed to ablate the sources of hormones capable of sustaining and stimulating the growth of breast cancer. These included ablation of the ovaries, adrenal glands and pituitary gland. Male and female hormones (androgens and estrogens) are still, although seldom, applied in the treatment of metastatic breast cancer and this decrease has undoubtedly contributed also the almost complete disappearance of some of the complications resulting from their use.

Newer chemotherapeutic agents, new combinations of the cytotoxic medications, different schedules applied to their administration, and new ways of using old medications, have greatly increased the therapeutic armamentarium used against this malignant disease.

All these developments and these successes have been built upon the information provided by those physicians who, in the past, had treated breast cancer with surgery alone but in the process had accumulated invaluable information about the biology and the course of that disease. It is the accumulation of such information that has made it possible to progress to the present day diagnostic and therapeutic programs. While the old surgeons have been profusely criticized for their radical approach to treatment they are the ones who established the base of today's knowledge and understanding of that cancer.

The diagnostic capabilities of the present day imaging equipment and of the new biological testing methods have rendered possible the much earlier detection of the spread of breast cancer. While the role of these diagnostic capabilities in prolonging survival is constantly being re-evaluated they have made possible the application treatment before the development of serious problems due to metastases.

Research into the genetic and other biological characteristics of breast cancer has opened new avenues for potential treatment. Immunotherapy and the combination of immunotherapy linked to chemotherapy as well as improvements in radiation technology are being designed to target more precisely the tumor cells while sparing normal tissues, in a way akin to the smart bombs of mechanical wars, homing in on their targets.

Genetic explorations of breast cancer tissue have already yielded some invaluable information about some of the genetic abnormalities that increase the risk of this tissue becoming cancerous long before that change happens. It is very probable that more genetic information will be forthcoming in the very foreseeable future. The developments in the science of genetics have opened the prospect of making it possible to recognize and then, eventually, possibly, to repair the genetic damage or abnormalities that cause certain cells to become cancerous and, by so doing, reverse that process.

While the many forms of interventions applied to the treatment of breast cancer have generally improved the course of this malignancy they have also been associated sometimes with an aftermath of long term damage to the health and well-being of the recipients of chemotherapy, other forms of systemic therapy or radiation therapy administered or applied at various times. In the future the application of new technologies, better equipment, better targeting of tumor cells with better preservation of the integrity of normal tissues will decrease the probability of treatment-induced problems. It is also anticipated that progress in understanding the biological processes that lead to the various forms of cellular damage may lead to the development of methods that will repair it.

Based upon observations of the ethnic lifestyle and dietary habits of large populations, studies of the environmental factors, among which exposure to some external factors added to the genetic information, have also revealed some of the processes that may result in an increased risk for developing that disease. In turn, this knowledge helps in the development of interventions or recommendations for lifestyle and dietary changes designed to decrease that risk.

The patient's personal wishes in terms of her life, as modified by both that illness and its treatment, have become important components of the therapeutic goals. Great progress has taken place in the understanding of the management of the many distressing symptoms of cancer. As a result of this, it has become possible to develop treatment programs directed specifically to the maintenance of a good quality to the life of those suffering with cancer at any stage of their disease. The concept of "quality of life" as part of the evaluation of the benefit of any treatment has also finally entered into the decision-making system of treatment planning. No longer is the illness the only target of the treatment. Quality of life has become one of the end points of any anti-cancer treatment and has in itself become a treatment goal.

A further look into the crystal ball of the future next leads us to foresee also a time not too far away when, to preventive methods already available, may be added newer, more specific, and more effective ones that will become applicable to rid all women of the fear of this devastating disease. Until then this goal will be approached either by protecting them from it, by curing it if it occurs anyway, or, failing this, by long term, new and more effective treatment. As in many chronic illnesses, such a treatment may prolong life to the point of approaching its normal span although without necessarily curing the illness itself, while, at the same time, maintaining all along a good quality of life throughout its course.

That crystal ball constantly generates hope.